Praise for the Author

"Sharon Moloney has long been dedicated to bringing forth the sacredness of women's bodies and the importance of female biology in personal identity and as a gift to the world — the gift of life. In a time when people are becoming more and more mechanized and detached from the body, this book brings us back to earth, reminding us we are part and parcel of nature."

> – Vicki Noble, artist, healer, teacher, author of *Shakti Woman* and *The Double Goddess* and co-creator of *Motherpeace Tarot Cards and Playbook.*

"Sharon Moloney has a wealth of knowledge and an impressive depth of understanding about the female body, developed over decades of ground-breaking work in both academic and practical contexts. In this illuminating book, she combines scientific research with the spiritual context of women's embodiment, offering the reader a profound awareness of what it means to be born female."

> – Lara Owen, author of *Her Blood Is Gold: Awakening to the Wisdom of Menstruation*.

"Sharon brings authenticity, wisdom, and power to her life-long exploration of the feminine, as a woman, therapist, mother and writer, and her sharing is generous and deeply nourishing for all of us."

> – Dr Sarah Buckley, author of *Gentle Birth, Gentle Mothering.*

D1571978

"From the first words of Sharon's Introduction, we know we are in safe hands. Her knowledge base covers feminist theories, as well as biological and spiritual perspectives. We know she will keep all these important facets of life as female in mind throughout her book. In the years I have known Sharon, I have been witness to her exquisite and meticulous scholarship, and her beauty of mind and heart which glows in her physical presence. Our conversations have given mutual strength as we each attend the embodiment of femaleness."

 – **Kaye Gersch, PhD, Jungian psychotherapist, clinical supervisor, couples therapist.**

"Sharon is highly educated in the fields of psychotherapy, human physiology (particularly of childbirth, menstruation and the stress response) and theology, including the teachings of diverse spiritual traditions. She is a gifted educator and researcher, and a wise counsellor for people from every walk of life, complemented by the wisdom of lived experience. Sharon is a Wise Woman in every sense of the word. She is diligent and creative, sober and joyful, irreverent and deeply respectful of the sacred, nurturing and assertive, wise and playful."

 – **Dr Mary Emeleus, GP, Grad Dip Rural MMH (Psychotherapy), FASPM.**

"I attended Sharon's focus group exploring women's thoughts about menstruation and their reproductive life as part of her Doctoral research. At the time I was peri-menopausal and dreading the years that lay ahead. The way Sharon discussed being a woman in that session completely flipped my thinking. I saw menopause to be a powerful and positive time in my life, the essence of validation of my reproductive life and my womanhood. This strongly influenced my understanding of the role that midwives play in educating, advocating and supporting women."

 – **Marie McAuliffe, midwife, senior lecturer and midwifery coordinator.**

"As a participant in Sharon's workshops, I have gained much insight, particularly as a midwife promoting normal physiological birth. The workshops assisted me to gain a better understanding of the paternalistic world women find themselves in, and the sexualisation of women to the detriment of how they perceive and value menstruation, pregnancy, birth and lactation. Sharon is making an incredible contribution to women and families."

 – Rosalind Lock, endorsed midwife and midwifery lecturer.

"Written with a soft and intuitive flair, this book aptly and magnetically draws the reader in deeper, unfolding its juiciness as each page turns. Uniquely, this go-to resource about Female Power is inclusive of all genders and provides an enlightening experience for sex educators and birthing professionals alike."

 – Alex Fox, sexological bodyworker, educator and pleasure coach.

Activate Your
Female Power

Dear Mary-Janet
Love your beautiful body.
It is truly sacred.
with love
Sharon
xx

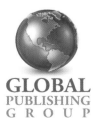

GLOBAL
PUBLISHING
GROUP

Global Publishing Group
Australia • New Zealand • Singapore • America • London

Activate Your Female Power

Reclaim Your Body, Fertility, Health, Happiness and Confidence as a Woman

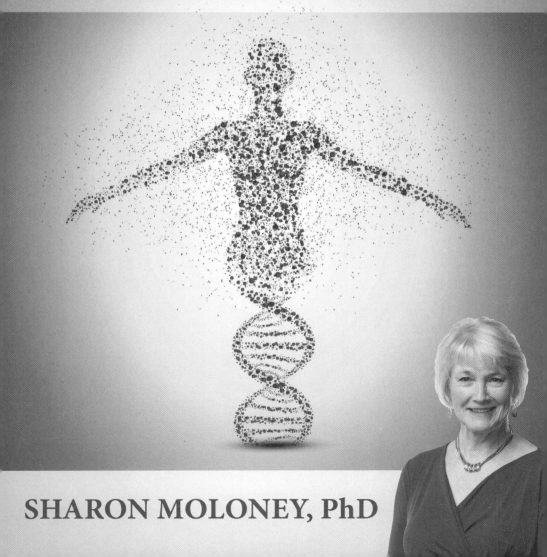

SHARON MOLONEY, PhD

First Edition 2018

 A catalogue record for this book is available from the National Library of Australia

Published by Global Publishing Group
PO Box 517 Mt Evelyn, Victoria 3796 Australia
Email info@GlobalPublishingGroup.com.au

Printed in China

For further information about orders:
Phone: +61 3 9739 4686 or Fax +61 3 8648 6871

Illustrations by Caitlin Moloney
E: caitlin.moloneyy@gmail.com

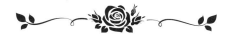

I dedicate this book to all the women of the world,
who are searching for their beauty and power,
and don't know where to find it.
May you discover it right there,
within your amazing bodies.

I also dedicate this book to Earth, our beautiful blue Planet,
who is so generous and abundant, and who now needs our
female leadership to show the way forward.

May we rise to the occasion with irrepressible
optimism and courage!

Acknowledgements

My first acknowledgement goes to my beloved husband and soul mate, Gerard, for his unfailing support and for being in the 'ship' of relationship with me. In addition to being my best friend, lover and loyal supporter, he has generously provided the practical means to enable me to dedicate myself to writing this book. Thank you, my love. His respectful maleness and our partnership inspire me to believe that equal relationships between women and men are possible.

I acknowledge my gifted daughter, Caitlin, who did the beautiful diagrams for this book, and fell down the rabbit hole with me into the bigger project about female biology as sacred. Caitlin, it means the world to me that you are on board and ready to take my work into the future.

I also acknowledge the spirit of my mother, who passed away many years ago and surprisingly showed up again during the writing of this book. Given our uneasy relationship during her lifetime, it's a gift to experience her support now.

I acknowledge Louise Hay's invaluable contribution in teaching me how to take charge of my mind. I thank the many people whose originality of thought has contributed to the ideas in this book; they are named in the references.

I am indebted to Sarah Buckley, Mary Emeleus, Alex Gardner, Kaye Gersch, Laura-Doe Harris and Lara Owen for reading various chapters of this book and offering invaluable refinements. Thank you dear friends.

My heartfelt thanks go to the team at Global Publishing Group for their constant encouragement and support, and especially to Darren Stephens, for his generosity and belief in me.

Bonus Offers

MP3 Recording: *Activate Your Female Power.*

This recording by Dr Sharon Moloney is designed to enable you to *Activate your Female Power.* Listen to the recording for at least 28 days to reprogram unhelpful beliefs about being female and to create a relationship of love with your body and the Earth. As you activate your female power, changes will begin happening inside you, as repressed energies are released, long-forgotten wisdoms wake up and dormant potentials are sparked into life.

E-Book: *Female Hormones*

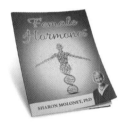

This e-book is a comprehensive guide to the mystical world of female hormones. In simple, easy-to-understand terms, we explore the principle and better known female hormones, oestrogen and progesterone, as well as the lesser known but equally significant role of testosterone. We look at the hormones made by the brain and the way they interact with the other hormones in a sophisticated feedback system. We briefly examine the hormones during pregnancy and the fascinating role of the placenta. We reflect on the fact that hormones are 'mind chemicals' that act on the brain and consequently play a vital role in shaping our consciousness, perceptions, moods, thought processes and spirituality.

Contents

Introduction 1

Section One – The Beginning of Life **15**

    Chapter One – Sex Determination 16

    Chapter Two – Sex Differentiation 27

Section Two – The Female Reproductive System **41**

    Chapter Three – The Holographic Template For Health 42

    Chapter Four – The Ovaries 48

    Chapter Five – The Oviducts Or Uterine Tubes 62

    Chapter Six – The Uterus 72

    Chapter Seven – The Vagina 93

    Chapter Eight – The Vulva 107

Section Three – The Blood Mystery **119**

    Chapter Nine – Menstruation 120

Conclusion **138**

About the Author **143**

Recommended Resources **145**

References **151**

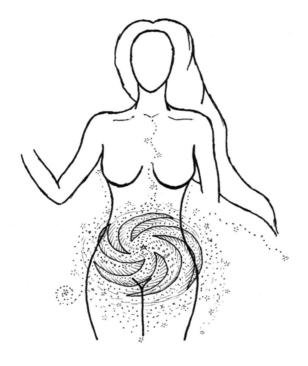

*"Within your physical body,
lie all the secrets and mysteries
of the Universe."*

Grandmother Sophia Thin Sticks.

Introduction

We have a secret in our culture. It's that women are strong and powerful - like the mother bear. A new mother will instinctively want to tear to shreds anything that threatens her baby. Any woman who endures the death of her baby is unbelievably strong. That same strength and power is also present in women who've never had children; it's a biological endowment that comes with being female. In the Western world, however, we live in a male-dominant culture, with a male deity and masculine ways of doing things as the norm, so we often don't recognise our female power and strength for what it is. And yet it's right there, inside our bodies, just waiting for us to claim it.

How we define something determines how we experience it. Menstruation is not meant to be an affliction, any more than birth is meant to be an ordeal. Yet for millions of women all around the world, that's how it is – in both domains. Contrary to what many people think, suffering through our female body processes is not what Nature intended. Quite the converse. As you'll discover through this book, female physiology is superbly designed. It is not, as we've been led to believe, inherently flawed, painful and destined to malfunction.

The perception of femaleness as a liability is a cultural myth that developed through thousands of years of forgetting the sacredness and potency of the female body. In many cultures around the world, from the ancient pre-patriarchal past right up to the present, women have experienced menstruation and giving birth as powerful, spiritual experiences that connect them to Nature, to their own authority and agency, to Earth and the Universe. You are entitled to experience that too. In fact, it's your birthright.

Attitude is everything. If you change your mind, you change what happens in your body. This is because the body is *in* the mind, like a fish is in water. By changing your beliefs, attitudes and feelings about your female body, you can modify your physiology for the better. Once you understand how to do this, it's entirely possible to transform your experience of femaleness into a source of pleasure, power and deep spiritual connection. This book is a map into that transformation.

Knowledge is power. So the more you know about the design of your female physiology, the more you can appreciate and align with its template for health, and the more you'll be inclined to change beliefs and practices that work against it. In the process, you'll access the elemental power that resides in the female body through our ability to menstruate, conceive and grow babies, birth them onto the Planet and feed them from our breasts. This elemental power is also present in women who have never borne children or who've had hysterectomies, simply by virtue of their femaleness.

A Note About Me

Ever since my first menstrual period, I have *loved* being female. It has filled me with wonder and delight. My first bleed was a spontaneous spiritual awakening that connected me intimately with Nature and the greater processes of Earth: the tides, the seasons and the phases of the moon. Inwardly I felt transformed in a deeply beautiful way.[1] This initiation profoundly shaped all my subsequent menstruations and the meaning I gave to the process, and the other female body experiences that followed. Because my menarche was such a blessing, my femaleness felt like a gift, an intimate share in Nature's power of creation.

How this book came to be written wasn't all light and roses however. In the years following my menarche, I grappled with being female in a very male world and nowhere was this more apparent than in the realm of spirituality. During my late 20s, I experienced a persistently strong spiritual calling that eventually led me to spend several years as a contemplative nun. Living within a patriarchal model of spirituality didn't work for me. My body succumbed and when I became ill, it was time to leave. Eighteen months later, when I married the love of my life and really wanted a child, there were problems. Here's what happened.

After months of chronic pelvic pain, I sought medical help and an ultrasound showed multiple swollen follicles, bulging like bunches of grapes from my ovaries. Medicine couldn't help, so I went to the library and got out all the books I could find on the anatomy and physiology of the female reproductive system. I spent hours making notes, drawing diagrams and figuring out how my female biology functioned, right down to the cellular level.

Sitting at my desk one day, I looked up from my notes, gazing into the trees outside... and the miraculous nature of what I was studying overwhelmed me. I saw that the female body is an exquisitely designed ecosystem, that the cells, tissues and organs are highly intelligent and responsive. I understood that energy is the primary reality and its signature is movement, transformation and health. I also realised that my body wasn't a badly designed machine that was randomly malfunctioning. My ovaries perfectly expressed the chronic stress, toxicity and spiritual imbalance that characterised my life at that time.

This 'aha' moment was the beginning of my recovery. I took full responsibility for restoring my health. I found a holistic doctor who practiced nutritional and herbal medicine; I eliminated all toxic chemicals from my home; I changed my diet to include more raw foods; I had regular kinesiology and acupuncture sessions; I found a therapist to support me through the emotional, psychological and spiritual changes. And most importantly, I began to really appreciate my body.

I realised the 'God' I'd been looking for in all the wrong places was right here under my nose. I discovered that female biology is both sacred and miraculous– a discovery that eventually became the topic of my doctoral research. About a year after this 'aha' moment, at the age of 40, I conceived and, nine months later, gave birth to my beautiful daughter.

Out of that adversity, this book was born and along with it, my path with heart. From then on, I decided to dedicate my life to raising awareness of the sacredness of the female body. When my daughter started kindergarten, I began writing up what I'd learned from my studies in order to make the information accessible to others. I kept the medical terminology, so people could understand their medical reports and doctors' language; I also found the Latin words had interesting meanings that helped describe an organ's function.

In the following chapters, I share this detailed information about female biology, using the same spiritual awareness that opened up for me as I studied it. This inner landscape is truly a playground of Spirit and if you open your mind and heart to that possibility, it will be a game-changer for you. Even if it's information you already know, be willing to see it through new eyes, and it will reward you deeply.

A Note on Feminism

Some feminists view focussing on female biology as 'essentialist', meaning that it's locating gender back in the body – sometimes a cardinal sin for contemporary feminist theory's orthodoxy, which maintains that gender is always socially constructed. Here's how I see it. Historically, feminists sought to minimise biological differences and emphasised the social construction of gender to secure equal treatment and pay in the workplace. While the demand for equal status in a male-dominant world was a necessary progression, it did not correct the imbalance between male and female energies in our world. And the notion that gender is purely a social construction ignores the specifics of the female body, like the needs of the menstrual cycle, physiological requirements for optimal birthing, or the female pattern of sexual arousal.

Many of the women I interviewed for my PhD described how the feminist insistence on equal status in a male world had failed to support their full humanity as *female*. As one participant noted, the insistence that we're all the same devalues women even more because "our differences seem to be worth so little". Another remembered that when she worked in the corporate world "the feminist idea of women being able to do everything seemed not to include mothering". Yet another participant spoke of feeling cheated by a feminism that had distanced itself from the body and how birthing her son awakened a deep grief about being so disconnected.

The omission of these central female experiences from the mainstream feminist agenda means that menstrual shame, fear of birth, birth trauma and women's sexual suppression continue. My participants' testimonies highlight the inadequacy of a feminist insistence that men and women are all the same, that our bodies are simply passive recipients of social conditioning. Something infinitely more mysterious and powerful than 'discourses' is evident in our female bodies, something capable of lighting us up and changing us to the roots of our being.

That 'something' needs a feminist framework to validate our life-changing experiences and enable us to positively understand and appreciate what we experience through our bodies, whether we have children or not. We need the solidarity of a collective that supports us to withstand the patriarchal pressures that undermine, suppress or even actively destroy those experiences. And we also need the backing of a political movement that fights to protect these uniquely precious dimensions of our lives. As feminist scholar Jo Murphy-Lawless noted:

> *"The idea of men embodying power is part of Western culture. It is the task of feminism ... to enable the pregnant and labouring woman to be defined as embodying an exceptional form of power, as she undergoes childbirth."* [2]

A feminist framework that *does* acknowledge this exceptional power is cultural feminism (aka spiritual feminism), which honours both the fertile Earthbody and the female body for their elemental life-giving powers. [3] Cultural feminism maintains that gender is comprised of biology *and* culture, not either or. It also claims that a *reciprocally rewarding* relationship exists between our female body and the Earthbody. This connection is what I spontaneously experienced during my menarche and as I discovered through my research, other women experience it too. That reciprocal relationship is available to any woman who wants to access it, including you. What's more, according to cultural feminism, the cosmological power residing in the female body holds the potential to change the world. And *that's* where we're going in this book!

A Note on Sexual Difference

Many Indigenous societies respect sex differences between women and men. In Western culture, we've forgotten this wisdom to our detriment. In our social context, women have adapted to their workplaces by adopting a masculine psychology, which is task-focussed, linear and goal-oriented. Many people see this *modus operandi* as the norm and our female bodies as irrelevant. Yet, as mammals, women have a cyclic physiology with a consistent need for down-regulation of the nervous system. The discrepancy between this mammalian need and the requirements of the workplace creates an inherent stress in the female body.

Femaleness is physiologically a very different mode of being to maleness. One of the most important contributions we can make as women is to understand and respect this difference. Many key activities associated with being female – lovemaking, conception, birthing, breastfeeding and the strong pair bonds of mother and baby– have a number one requirement of SAFETY! To conceive, I must feel safe. To open up and birth, I must feel safe. To allow the milk let-down reflex, I must feel safe. To surrender to the pleasure of my body in lovemaking, I must feel safe.

Many women don't feel safe and don't even realise that they don't feel safe because their chronic hyper-vigilance from living a masculine lifestyle has become so normal. In effect, they've forgotten they are female. When women are expected – and expect themselves – to be just like men in order to succeed, it exacts a heavy penalty, especially in their reproductive health. If this is you, don't despair. You can dismantle that hyper-vigilance by learning how to access your deep relaxation response. If you want to conceive and it's not happening, regularly practicing deep relaxation really helps because your body receives the message that it's safe and now is a good time to conceive. [4]

On Being Female

What does it mean to be female? Is it simply a random event, an accident of nature with no real significance? Or does it have meaning and purpose? We're going to spiral around these questions throughout this book. Some of the things being female means are:

- an X-X combination of sex chromosomes inside the nucleus of every cell of your body

- the presence of female sex hormones during our early weeks as an embryo that appear to influence the pattern by which our brain develops

- a cyclic fertility pattern with fluctuations and the ebb and flow of cyclic processes

- the ability to participate intimately in the incarnation of another human being during pregnancy, to give birth and then feed that baby from your breasts

- a subjective experience of the female body with its unique architecture that's designed for boundary-penetration

- a distinctly female mode of perception, with its own ways of knowing, terms of reference and composition of meanings

- an experience of spirituality thoroughly grounded in our bodies and our physiological processes

Femaleness permeates our existence from the cellular level up, so our subjective experience as human beings is different from that of maleness. Why is that so important? Because as we all know, our world is wildly out of balance in its male/female energies and it needs our conscious *female* presence to correct that imbalance. To show up in that capacity, we need to be at home in the rhythms of our female bodies, not acting like men.

I use the word 'female' because of its biological significance. The dictionary defines 'female' as: "*of the offspring bearing sex.*"[5] The word has its origins in the Latin 'femina', meaning woman, of which 'femella' is the diminutive form. The root meaning is *"she who suckles"* (from the Latin 'felare', *to suckle young*), so as humans, we belong to the family of animals who feed their young from their breasts, and this mammalian link is crucial when it comes to fertility and birthing.

To fully grasp the magnificence of being female, we need to consider our nature as spiritual beings and the historical context in which biology became separated from spirituality. In the next section, I provide some of that background, which may seem like a philosophical tangent, but I promise you, it's completely relevant. Context is everything, so come with me because what you'll learn will enable you to appreciate the magic of where we're going inside our amazing bodies.

Our Humanity as Spiritual Beings

To me, a human being is a luminous animal, a creature of spirit rooted in matter and the earth. How does our existence bridge these two dimensions? How are we both mortal and immortal? In his book *Radical Forgiveness,* Colin Tipping describes how we're made with a foot in each camp: one in the physical world, which we know through our five senses, and one in spiritual reality, which we know inwardly through our spirit. What connects the two is our soul.

> *"While being fully grounded in the World of Humanity, we are connected to the World of Divine Truth through our soul ... Our soul carries a vibration that resonates with the World of Divine Truth."*[6]

The word vibration reflects the discovery that life energy is dynamic, for example, human DNA vibrates at a rate of 52–78 gigahertz (billions of cycles) per second.[7] When we vibrate at slower frequencies, we become immersed in the world of humanity and five sensory reality, whereas at higher frequencies, the world of spirit is more accessible to us. Our human predicament sees us constantly moving between these two poles, as depicted in the following diagram.

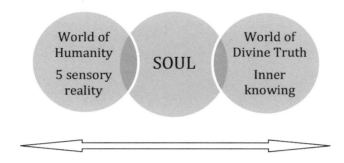

What's important to understand is that the world of humanity and the world of divine truth co-exist in the present: *"These existential realms differ not in terms of place or time but solely in their vibrational level."*[8] While the conventional religion I grew up with depicted human beings as having occasional spiritual experiences, with eternal life seen as a superannuation after death, the above model depicts us as primarily *spiritual* beings, having a human experience. What's the relevance of this to gender? Our sex profoundly shapes how we, as spiritual beings, experience being human. Female spirituality can make the connection with our immortal self quite differently from male spirituality because of our unique capacity to menstruate, grow babies, birth them and breastfeed. When male models of spirituality are assumed as the norm, we can entirely miss the power of our own experiences.

A Note about Biology

Hidden deep inside our female bodies is a truly remarkable spirituality that most of us know nothing about. Our physiology holds unique opportunities to deepen our connection with the world of Spirit. Our biology is also a metaphor for the rest of our lives, as my ovaries taught me. Like a mirror, it accurately reflects our history. Medical intuitive Caroline Myss describes how it does this:

> *"All our thoughts, regardless of their content, first enter our systems as energy. Those that carry emotional, mental, psychological or spiritual energy produce biological responses that are then stored*

in our cellular memory. In this way our biographies are woven into our biological systems, gradually, slowly, every day."[9]

Our biography thus becomes our biology. Our bodies carry all the stored memories, emotions, beliefs, attitudes and vibrations of our personal history, lineage and culture, which can have dramatic consequences for our health, fertility and spirituality.

The Separation of Biology and Spirit

In Western culture, biology and spirituality have typically been seen as separate and unrelated domains. When I looked up the word 'spiritual' in the dictionary, I found this definition: "Relating to the spirit or soul and *not to physical nature or matter*".[10] This definition perfectly expresses our cultural separation of matter and spirit, and also a patriarchal view of spirituality.

There are historical reasons dating back to the Enlightenment that help to explain this separation. During the seventeenth century, René Descartes was formulating his philosophy of science amidst the turmoil of the Reformation. To avoid the theological disputes of the time, Descartes based his description of reality on the separate entities of: God – the World – the human person.[11] Newtonian physics followed suit, based on the assumption that the world could be described without reference to God or human beings. The philosophy of science that developed out of this worldview thus separated body and spirit into two mutually exclusive domains.[12]

Scientists came to view the material world, including Earth and the human body, as a multitude of different objects assembled into a huge machine.[13] This mechanistic worldview underpinned Newtonian physics and the Enlightenment project of exploring and conquering the natural world. 'Reality' was seen as objectively observable, derived solely from the senses and based on fixed universal laws of cause and effect that existed independently of human consciousness. Human beings were seen as rational individuals governed by social laws.

This paradigm allowed scientists (and everyone else) to treat the material world as dead, unspiritual and completely disconnected from themselves. The notion of the mechanical universe and the body as a machine carried over into most scientific disciplines and became entrenched in our major institutions like hospitals, universities, public services and churches. In the latter half of the last century, we started seeing the devastating global consequences of this worldview and its alienation from Nature. Industrial exploitation of Earth's natural resources, pollution, species extinction, deforestation, nuclear accidents and most notably climate change are some of the compelling consequences now confronting us.

Fast forward three centuries and science itself now confirms the inseparability of matter and spirit, a theme we explore further in Chapter Three. As I experienced in my 'aha' moment, biology and spirit are one and the same. Our body processes at the cellular level are Life Force energy in action. Matter does miraculous things under the quickening impulse of Spirit. This is true in a uniquely powerful way in the female body because of our capacity to conceive, grow and birth new human life – even if we never take that journey.

Female Spirituality

What does it mean spiritually to experience femaleness? Pondering this question led me to reflect on my own experience - on what it feels like within myself to have the soft roundness of breasts; to look out at the world through my female eyes, and interpret what I see, hear, smell, taste and touch through my female mind; to have a vaginal opening penetrate my pelvic floor and the open wetness of female genitals; to be penetrated by another person during lovemaking and experience prolonged waves of orgasmic pleasure; to know the red richness of menstruation each month; to conceive, grow and then birth a new human being, and to suckle that baby from my breasts; to feel my biology as a partnership with Spirit; to experience the cosmological power of my body as an intimate connection with Earth and the Universe.

These female experiences have profound meaning and significance. Ultimately, they are the embodiment of a unique spirituality. In our very architecture, we are designed as portals to Spirit. So much female body experience involves boundary penetration, from inside and outside: sexual intercourse, menstruation, birth and lactation. As Sylvia Brinton Perera observed: *"This penetration is analogous to the soul's penetration by the divine, "*a capacity based not on passivity, but an active willingness to receive. [14] This relationship potential, which occurs through our bodies and enables us to co-create with Spirit, in turn, generates a unique form of leadership. Referring to the female experience of gestation, birth and lactation, Sallie McFague notes:

"This experience in most animals, including human beings, engenders not attributes of weakness and passivity, but qualities contributing to the active defence of the young so that they may not only exist but be nourished and grow. Whatever thwarts such fulfilment is fought, often fiercely, as mother bears and tigers amply illustrate...Those who produce life have a stake in it and will judge, often with anger, what prevents its fulfilment." [15]

The ferocity of the mother bear is a force of Nature to which we are privy through our mammalian heritage. Being female endows us with a biological leadership which, if we're willing to unleash it, becomes a fierce determination to safeguard *all* life forms on the Planet.

Commit to the process

Research has shown that in traditions where women's bodies are honoured and respected, the Earthbody is also honoured and respected. [16] Earth is the macrocosm of which we are the microcosm. In our culture, *it has to start with us* - loving our bodies and respecting them as sacred, so we can teach the rest of the culture what this looks like and how to do it. When enough of us do this, our collective 'mother bear' ferociousness will insist that Earth be respected as the living, breathing, intelligent Being she is. This has to be our top priority because we've already gone past a tipping point that's irrevocably altered many of the major life support systems of our Planet, threatening not only our survival but that of many other species.

So I invite you to commit to the process that's offered in this book and engage with the material. Read it reflectively and let the information seep into your bones. Buy a journal and give yourself time to write in it. Explore the questions and suggestions at the end of each chapter and jot down any insights or feelings you notice. If you like drawing, sketch something to express your responses. Create your own affirmations and sacred rituals. Make your engagement with this book a commitment to honour yourself as a sacred female being, with your own unique contribution to make at this time and place.

In addition, you can deepen your transformation by downloading my MP3 recording *Activate Your Female Power*, freely available from the website (www.ActivateYourFemalePower.com) and listen to it daily for 28 days. This recording is designed to reprogram your subconscious mind by activating the sacred power inside your body and giving you a process to take ownership of it.

During this process, your relationship with your body, and consequently the Earthbody, will grow stronger. You may find an increase of energy running through your body, more strength in your muscles, organs and mind, greater peace and self-acceptance in your heart, hope for the future and the sheer joy of being alive in your wonderful female body. You may also find that your experiences of menstruation, birth, breastfeeding and sexuality have greater depth, meaning and pleasure.

The book is divided into three sections. In Section One, we look at the miraculous processes of sex determination and sex differentiation to understand how we actually began life as female. Section Two begins with the holographic template for health, followed by a guided tour through all the astounding organs in the female reproductive system. In Section Three, we begin exploring the Blood Mystery of menstruation, which is a bridge into my second book, *Following the Menstrual Flow: Through Menarche, Birth and Menopause*. Each section builds on the previous one, though you can pick the book up and dip into it however you like.

Researching this book drew me unavoidably into a study of aspects of maleness too. Along with the differences of each sex, I discovered some surprising similarities. I discovered, for instance, that for the first eight weeks of life from conception through the embryonic stage, we are neither definitively male nor female – we are simply human. Let's now explore this common humanity, as we look in more detail at the process of sex determination and how we all began life from a common embryonic foundation.

Section One

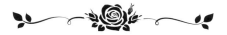

The Beginning of Life

Chapter One

❦

Sex Determination

Did you ever stop to reflect on how you began to incarnate onto this Planet as a female? Your own conception and morphology into a female body was quite a momentous journey with many twists and turns, and some potentially perilous transitions. It's not a given that what begins the process will end in new human life. As many as 40% of pregnancies miscarry in the first week after conception.[1] And it's not a simple 1 plus 1 equals 2. What actually determines whether that egg and sperm will go on to become a new individual is the *vertical energy coming down to connect with the physical substance that's been opened by fertilisation.*[2] When it does, then we have ignition! From that moment on, there is a new organism which is largely self-determining.

The organism is the primary reality, not the cells. Philosophically this is a very different perspective to the old paradigm, in which the organism arose out of the cells, like a house made of bricks. As embryologist Jaap van der Wal[3] observed, the primary entity of living nature is the *organism* and this organism is a dynamic process, out of which different parts emerge. Ponder this before we move on because it makes all the difference to how you'll think about cells in the rest of the book. *The organism is the primary entity and the cells are governed by the intelligence of the organism.* Basically, van der Wal is saying that we are an individual wholeness from the very beginning, rather than a collection of parts. Got that? Good, now let's move onto the cells.

To truly appreciate how we began life as female, we need to scale down our perspective to the smallest living units inside our bodies, the cells, because it's from this basic cellular level that we differ as male and female. Taking a microscopic look at life inside the cell gives us important

---

insights into how and why this difference occurs. While the next few paragraphs might seem a bit like your high school biology class, stay with it because we'll build on this information in the really interesting bits to follow and it will be worth it.

Inside the nucleus of every cell (except red blood cells which don't have a nucleus) are long bumpy threads of **chromatin** (*'coloured substance'*) which carry our genetic inheritance – deoxyribonucleic acid or **DNA**. These lumpy strands of DNA provide the coded instructions for directing the activities inside our cells. A **gene** is simply a segment of DNA that encodes a specific cell function, and all the cells in our body carry the same genes.

Normally the chromatin threads inside the nucleus lie entwined, like a skein of wool. Then when the cell prepares to divide and reproduce itself, a marvellous reorganisation occurs. (Figure 1.1) Prompted by the intelligence of the organism, the chromatin threads coil and condense, lining themselves up into compact rod-shaped pairs that are now called **chromosomes** (*'coloured bodies'*).

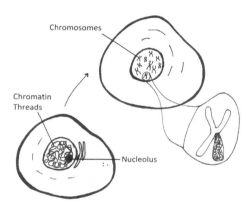

Figure 1.1

This ingenious move protects the delicate chromatin strands from breaking or getting tangled. Within the chromosomes, the DNA then cleverly arranges itself into the famous 'double helix' formation, resembling a spiral staircase. (Figure 1.2)

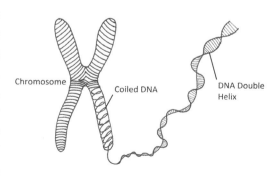

Figure 1.2

During this process of cell division, 23 pairs of chromosomes line up, one half of the pair inherited from our mother, the other from our father, making 46 in total. One pair, the sex chromosomes, contains the genetic inheritance that determines our sex: either an XX combination which is female, or an XY combination which is male. (Figure 1.3) The mother's egg can contribute only an X chromosome, while the father's sperm can contribute either another X chromosome, resulting in a female, or a Y chromosome resulting in a male.

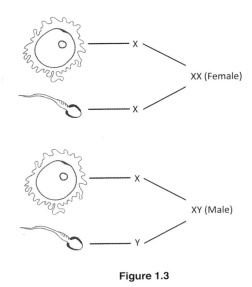

Figure 1.3

Under a microscope, the X chromosome is much larger than the Y chromosome and contains more genes. The Y chromosome (so called because it actually resembles the letter Y) contains a vital gene known as sex-determining region Y or SRY. It seems this gene is responsible for the initiation of male development. *Without this gene, female development occurs.*

Just think about that. It requires the presence of an additional factor, the SRY gene, for maleness to develop. This means that the default setting is actually *femaleness*. This biological fact deserves closer scrutiny. Symbolically, it represents a complete reversal of the creation mythology many of us grew up with – the story of Adam and Eve, in which femaleness derived from maleness. In the Book of Genesis, we read that Adam was lonely without a helpmate, so God fashioned him a woman. The story goes like this:

> *"So the Lord God caused a deep sleep to fall upon the man, and while he slept took one of his ribs and closed up its place with flesh; and the rib which the Lord God had taken from the man he*

made into a woman and brought her to the man. Then the man said: 'This at last is bone of my bones and flesh of my flesh; she shall be called Woman, because she was taken out of Man.'" (Genesis 2:21–23)[4]

For millennia, this mythological casting of the first human being as male has left woman as the afterthought, a helpmate to comfort and support the principal actor on life's stage. According to this origin story, maleness is the original human form, with femaleness a derivative. The legacy of the cultural mindset of woman as secondary and 'other' persists to this day because a culture's origin story is absorbed deep into the subconscious mind as a 'truth'.

We now know that not only is this presumption unfounded; it is biologically inaccurate. Femaleness is the basic human template, from which maleness deviates under the influence of the SRY gene. It's not simply the XY chromosome combination that guarantees male development. We know this because if the SRY gene is for some reason absent, then even though an XY combination is present, a female will develop. So take this important piece of information on board. You are not secondary to anyone; you are the original.

The chromosomal differences between the two sexes are encapsulated by Dr Irene Elia:

"Although it is the X-chromosome in double dose that is the signature of every mammalian female, it is not exclusively devoted to female sex determination. In fact, in humans, the traits that make a female female seem to be scattered over all her 23 chromosome pairs."[5]

By contrast:

"The small Y-chromosome, which is the signature of all mammalian males, carries almost no traits. The only known Y-linked trait, of the more than two thousand known human genetic traits, is the H-Y antigen trait. This antigen sticks to the surfaces of all male cells and causes the embryonic gonad to become a testicle. The only other trait that is Y-linked in some human groups is that

for hairy ear rims! Although the Y-chromosome is not a big trait carrier, it is vital to male differentiation of the embryo." [6]

As we saw earlier, only sperm cells carry the deciding factor in sex determination. During the 1960s, two different types of sperm cells were discovered: larger, more oval-shaped ones carrying the X chromosome and smaller, round-headed ones which carry the Y chromosome. The X chromosome sperm appeared hardier and able to survive longer in the naturally acidic environment of the vagina, while the Y chromosome ones appeared to swim faster than 'female' sperm in the more alkaline secretions around the time of ovulation. These differences gave rise to the theory that timing intercourse could influence the sex of the baby. Sex on the day of ovulation would enhance the chance of conceiving a son, while sex 2 or 3 days before ovulation would increase the odds of a daughter. Although research studies haven't substantiated the theory, there's some anecdotal evidence to support this idea.

Unlike other cells, **gametes** or sex cells (sperm and egg) contain only 23 chromosomes instead of the usual 46, so when they unite with each other at fertilisation, they come to their full complement. In all other body cells during cell division, the 23 pairs of chromosomes split, and each half undergoes an exact replication of DNA. In this way all the genetic material is perfectly preserved with its unique sequence of information. The identical sets of chromosomes then separate to form the nuclei of two daughter cells, each with 46 chromosomes. (Figure 1.4) Once the separation is complete, the chromosomes uncoil again and return to their original skein-like chromatin form. This complex and mysterious process is called **mitosis** (Greek mitos– *'thread'*).

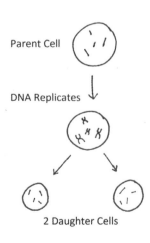

Parent Cell

DNA Replicates

2 Daughter Cells

Figure 1.4

Because sperm and egg cells need only half the number of chromosomes, they undergo an even more complex form of division, wherein they divide not once, but twice. For the egg, after each of these divisions, only one cell retains the substance, while the other half (called a polar body) disintegrates. For the sperm, all four offspring of this division go on to become sperm cells.

This process of **meiosis** (Greek meioun–'*to diminish*') ensures that when the sex cells fuse with each other at fertilisation, the outcome will be a completely new and original pairing of 46 chromosomes, containing all the genetic material needed for a unique human being. (Figure 1.5) Meiosis also accounts for a huge genetic variation in daughter cells, whereas mitosis ensures exact genetic copies.

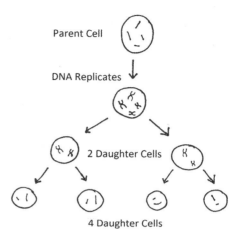

Figure 1.5

From this summary, we can see that sex determination – whether a male or a female is conceived – begins with the magical moment of fertilisation, when the two parent cells fuse together opening up a new possibility. In reality, this is not so much a moment, as a sophisticated, complex and miraculous process. From the sperm's perspective, it's a long journey of attraction to the powerful chemical signals radiating from the egg. From the egg's perspective, it's pure magnetism!

Considering that approximately 500 million sperm are present in one ejaculation, you might think that was an over-supply. However there's a good reason for this proliferation. Of those 500 million sperm, millions leak away from the vagina almost straight away. Unless the vagina and cervix are alkaline (as they are around the time of ovulation), most sperm are unable to penetrate the cervix and many of those that do, are dispersed throughout the womb cavity. Of the millions of sperm ejaculated, it's estimated that only a few thousand or less actually reach the egg.

When first ejaculated, sperm are unready to fertilise the egg because of the tough helmet-like structure, the **acrosome,** (Greek ákros – *'topmost'*) covering the outer membrane of the sperm head. (Figure 1.6) Consequently, sperm need to undergo a

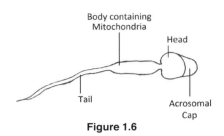

Figure 1.6

'capacitation' process that releases their fertilising powers. Here we see a mating dance, a dialogue between sperm and egg, in which our combined fertility collaborates beautifully. Fertile secretions in the cervix, uterus and tubes gradually ripen the sperm's acrosome membranes by depleting the cholesterol that maintains their toughness. This ripening can take up to eight hours, so although sperm may arrive in the vicinity of the egg within a short space of time, they must wait around, so to speak, before any chance of union can occur.

Meanwhile, the egg cell released during ovulation makes its way very slowly down the uterine tubes. At this stage, it's called an **oocyte** (from oogenesis – *'the beginning of an egg'*). It is surrounded by two protective layers beautifully named: the **zona pellucida** (*'transparent belt'*), and outside this, the **corona radiata** (*'radiating crown'*). (Figure 1.7) Experiments have shown that sperm find their way to the egg by responding to its scent, even when it's been heavily diluted. When the sperm reach the egg's vicinity, they become visibly excited and frenzied, thrashing and spinning in circles.

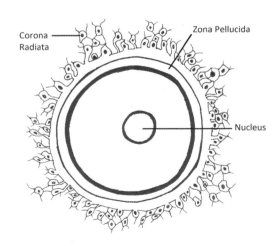

Figure 1.7

Photos of the oocyte taken with an electron microscope reveal a majestic translucent sphere that looks for all the world like a planet. When I first saw these photos, they reminded me of the pictures of our beautiful blue Earth taken from space. Fulsome and grand, the oocyte's sheer volume and mass convey substance and clout. It's the most substantial cell in our bodies, dwarfing every other cell. In its structure, function and activity, the egg cell displays amazing powers of creativity and resourcefulness. It is quite literally a powerhouse, indeed the repository of an exceptionally spiritual power. (The oocyte is explored in greater detail in Chapter Four: The Ovaries.)

Up until recently, the process of fertilisation was described through a male lens of intrepid, aggressive sperm heroically seeking out a passive 'damsel in distress'.[7] Recent research dispels this gender stereotyping by showing a mutual exchange between sperm and egg. For example, substances released by the egg both guide and activate the sperm, and in response, sperm release proteins that help them stick to the egg's surface.[8] A chemical produced in the egg cell (as well in the follicle that housed it and the womb lining), has a specific receptor for it in the head of the sperm. Receptors are like locks and when the key goes into the lock, reactions occur. This mechanism keeps the sperm locked onto the egg's surface until the cellular membranes between the two have time to dissolve.

Philosophers of old (St Thomas Aquinas among them) believed that sperm contained all that was needed to generate new human life. The female contribution was thought to be simply a womb in which to incubate and grow the miniature human being believed to inhabit the sperm. These misconceptions could not be further from the truth. In reality, the egg contains the vast bulk of the raw material needed for the cell processes after fertilisation. It actively orchestrates those cell processes with information encrypted not only in its nuclear DNA but also inside the abundance of mitochondria in its cytoplasm. Mitochondria are the cell's powerhouses, little organelles that take in nutrients and convert them to energy. Far from being a mere 'oven' in which to cook the embryo, the egg cell is the provider of the very stuff from which the cells of the new individual take their substance. More about this later!

When the pool of sperm reaches the egg, chemistry reigns supreme in a remarkable phenomenon known as the **acrosomal reaction**. (Figure 1.8) Once the sperm cells are locked on to the egg's leathery zona pellucida, another mating dance begins. A special protein in the zona acts upon the sperm and in return, their hyperactivity, which includes whipping tail movements and sideways swinging motions of their heads, continues the release of digestive enzymes. Secretions from hundreds of sperm together produce enough enzymes to clear a pathway to the egg's surface. At this point, a single sperm finally makes contact with the egg's membrane, and egg and sperm membranes fuse. The cosmos holds its breath!

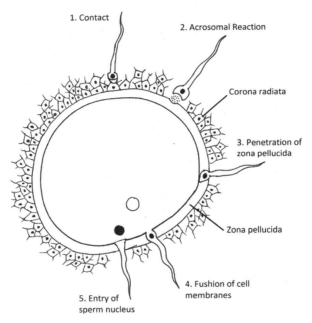

1. Contact
2. Acrosomal Reaction
Corona radiata
3. Penetration of zona pellucida
Zona pellucida
4. Fushion of cell membranes
5. Entry of sperm nucleus

Figure 1.8

The egg's response to this contact is electric – literally! Its outer membrane firstly depolarizes, an electrical event which prevents other sperm from penetrating. The membrane then floods with water and swells, detaching other sperm still in contact with its outer layers. The sperm then turns 180 degrees so the posterior part of its head now becomes absorbed by the egg's cytoplasm. Simultaneously it sheds its tail and midsection, as they've accomplished their task of propelling the sperm to its destination.

All that's now left of the sperm is a dense package of DNA, the nuclear remains of what began as a complete cell. As the remaining head enlarges, it begins migrating towards the centre of the egg, a process which can take up to 12 hours.

Finally the two pronuclei (with half the number of chromosomes) meet near the egg's centre, their nuclear membranes fuse and their precious genetic cargo now merges into the full complement of 46 chromosomes needed for new human life. This is the moment when 'ignition' becomes possible. The stage is set; the invitation is there for the vertical energy to come on in. The culmination of such an epic and magnificently orchestrated journey seems inadequately conveyed by the term 'fertilisation'.

This moment remains one of our most mysterious life processes. We know the intimate details of what happens when these two nuclei fuse together. We can describe the chemistry, the electrical activity, the cellular physiology; we can even replicate the process in a petri dish. Yet for all that, this miraculous moment when another human being begins its life remains shrouded in mystery. It is infinitely more than the sum of its parts. As van der Wal[9] puts it, when spirit and matter meet, you have life; when spirit and matter separate, you have death. The incarnation of another soul onto the Planet is a profoundly spiritual occurrence, in which spirit transforms matter. When a new individual begins this process, the whole universe has to shift to accommodate the change.

In the very instant of this consummation, the fertilised egg begins to divide in two, the first two cells of what will eventually become a unique human being. If the fertilising sperm was a Y-bearer, a boy will have been conceived. If it was an X-bearer, a girl will be on her way and we have the beginnings of a new incarnation of femaleness – an identical process, regardless of gender, whose outcome is determined solely by the presence or absence of a miniscule particle of DNA – an X or a Y chromosome.

In reflecting upon this miraculous process, we can see that even at this most elementary level, the female sex cell requires and orchestrates a boundary penetration by the sperm, in order to fulfil its destiny. As we shall see in subsequent chapters, this phenomenon of boundary penetration recurs so often in our biology, it could be described as the quintessential female experience. Without that boundary penetration, the egg will die within 24–48 hours, as will the sperm.

Genetically speaking then, what distinguishes female from male is minute but profound; it is simply the difference of one chromosome. However this one chromosome makes all the difference. It contains the genetic instructions for either female development or male development and it's present within every cell in our bodies. And when you consider that these cells comprise all of our organs, glands, muscles, skin, bones, and brains, then it's obvious that what seems so minute a difference, has profound consequences indeed.

Reflection

What I now know about beginning life as a female that I didn't know before is…

What I most love and appreciate about beginning life as female is…

When I reflect on this information, what strikes or moves me is…

Affirmation

Beginning life as female is a mystery that fills me with pride.

Suggestion

Look at the pictures of the ovum, Earth, the sperm and the embryo in the middle section of this book. Gaze at the images with an open heart; let them speak to you. As you view these pictures, consider what's meant by the 'vertical energy coming in' to the fertilised egg and how the female gamete acts like a lightning rod for Spirit. Draw a picture that depicts this event.

Chapter Two

Sex Differentiation

Whilst sex determination occurs at the very moment of conception, the process by which the tiny embryo becomes either female or male – sex differentiation – takes place some weeks later. Despite the male/female gender divide we have all been taught to believe is normal, this differentiation process is far from straightforward or mutually exclusive. It involves three distinct windows of development – the gonads, the genitals and the brain – each of which brings ample opportunity for variations on the theme. We now know that there's a spectrum of gender, rather than a simple male/female binary. Individuals who identify as non-binary, intersex or transgender are showing us that the differentiation process can result in an outcome that fits neither gender category and that this diversity is normal and what you would expect from such a mutable process. More on this later!

For the purposes of this book, my focus is on the differentiation that results in femaleness. The vast leap from single-celled fusion into a recognisably human form unfolds during the furious activity of the embryonic phase. At the end of this time by week eight, all the major organs are in place and functioning in their rudimentary form and the tiny embryo, which is only about an inch long, is visibly male or female. This journey involves some unexpected twists and turns, fascinating facts and complex scientific information, so stay with me through it because you'll gain a wonderful expansive view by the end.

Fertilisation to Implantation

To arrive at 'embryo-hood', we must first backtrack to the moment of fertilisation when sperm and egg unite in the outer third of the uterine tube. The luminous sphere, now called a **zygote** ('*union*' or '*joined together*') begins a process of cell division as it travels slowly towards the uterus. (Figure 2.1) In an intriguing about-face, the same fluid which previously swept the sperm along the tube towards the

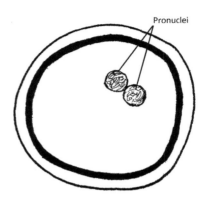

Figure 2.1

egg, now reverses its flow in response to the maternal hormones, much like the ebb and flow of the tides. I find it amazingly clever that the tubes know how to do this! The anemone-like cilia lining the tubes sweep their tendrils creating a current that swirls the sphere towards the uterine cavity, a journey lasting three to four days.

Around 72 hrs after fertilisation, there are 12 to 16 identical cells and the mulberry-shaped formation is quaintly named a **morula** (*'mulberry'*). As the morula travels along the tube, its cells continue to divide, each one becoming progressively smaller, so that the entire mass still remains encased within the now stretched outer shell of the zona. (Figure 2.2) By day four, the morula, which is about

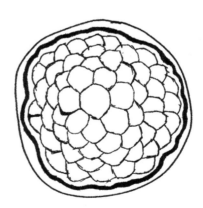

Figure 2.2

100 cells, drifts into the uterus where it floats freely for a couple of days. As it floats, two significant events occur. Firstly, the zona, the tough outer membrane which protected the inner cell mass in transit and prevented an untimely implantation in the tube, begins to hatch. And simultaneously,

the cells within the sphere, for the first time, begin to differentiate in readiness for implantation.

At this point, the morula becomes a **blastocyst,** (*'hollow bag of germ cells'*) so-called because it develops a central fluid-filled cavity. (Figure 2.3) At the same time, the cells now differentiate into two distinct groups: an outer **trophoblast** (*'nourishment generator'*) which goes on to develop into the placenta and membranes, and an inner mass of cells, which becomes the **embryo** (*'teem within'*).

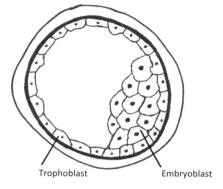

Trophoblast   Embryoblast

Figure 2.3

This intelligent little organism then discerningly tests the womb lining to assess its readiness for nesting. If it finds the right chemical signals high in the uterus, it will implant there. If not, it floats to a lower level looking for a more welcoming spot. This phenomenon may explain why women practicing deep relaxation have higher rates of successful implantation during IVF.[1] From the blastocyst's perspective, a womb lining saturated with endorphins released during deep relaxation is a welcoming place to burrow in, whereas a lining full of stress hormones will give off a very different signal. Regularly practicing deep relaxation during IVF is one of several ways a woman can enhance her chances of successful implantation.

When the blastocyst finds its preferred spot, it burrows into the thick, red, velvety womb lining, sinking down tendrils like tree roots. (We cover this process in more detail in Chapter Six.) As this burrowing-in process penetrates the womb lining, there's sometimes a small show of blood during implantation. Once hatched from its shell and snuggled in to the endometrium, there's no stopping the blastocyst! Within a day, cell numbers proliferate rapidly from 120 to 1000 and a day later, to 10,000.[2]

What follows is an explosion of activity with ongoing cell divisions and streaming migrations of cells, all of which differentiate into their specialised forms, organising themselves into a wondrously orchestrated master plan. The fine details of the individuality for the new organism are encapsulated in the unique genetic code embedded in the DNA within each cell nucleus. This phenomenal process, known as **organogenesis**, bears testimony to the cellular intelligence within us. As Elaine Marieb observed: *"It is truly amazing how much organogenesis occurs in such a short time in such a small amount of living matter."*[3]

Embryonic Phase

So begins the embryonic phase of the new individual's life, lasting from implantation on about day seven after fertilisation and continuing for roughly eight weeks. By the end of this time, all the major organs and systems are in place, though they are structurally and functionally still in their rudimentary stages. The heart has begun beating, the first brain waves are evident, sex differentiation has occurred and the body looks distinctly human. (Figure 2.4) Let's now take a look at those three windows of development that bring about the differentiation into female or male.

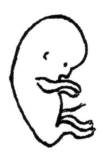

Figure 2.4

1) Differentiation of the gonads

Sex differentiation is completed right towards the end of the embryonic period, a process that begins in earnest at about week five when the **gonads** (ovaries or testes) begin their development. At first there's neither ovary nor testis, but a bi-potential **gonadal ridge**, which could develop either way. There are also *two* sets of tubes laid down; the embryo has *both* sets of ducts, one that could become female, the other male.

At this stage, the embryo is said to be sexually indifferent because *both the gonadal ridge and the ducts are structurally identical and can develop either way.* Just ponder the significance of that for a moment. I still vividly remember the excitement I felt upon learning those facts for the first time. What it means is that all of us, male and female, begin life on common ground, not just metaphorically but literally. Our embryonic forms are identical. We are *biologically the same before we become different*. Now why should that be of significance?

In our gender identification, we tend to think of ourselves as having always been female or male, right from the beginning of our existence. This belief gives us the impression that 'I am completely different from you because you are male and I am female'. Discovering that we were the same before we were different enables us to appreciate our common humanity. Yes, we *are* different and our differences need to be respected. Yet embryologically, o*ur sameness preceded our difference!*

What's more, with the possession of both rudimentary duct systems, we have also experienced the potential for opposite-sex development. In Taoism, the yin/yang symbol depicts the balanced wholeness of yin (female) and yang (male) energies, each containing aspects of the other inside themselves. In the West since Carl Jung, it's been widely accepted that psychologically we each have feminine and masculine aspects within ourselves. Little did we know that this was true in a very literal sense when we were only six-week-old embryos!

Amazingly, what determines the direction of our sexual development is the next generation of sex cells. To follow this process, we need to backtrack again to the time just after implantation when the membranes develop, which go onto become the amniotic sac and umbilical cord. Along with the amnion and cord, a **yolk sac** also develops, which hangs from the surface of the embryo. (Figure 2.5) The yolk sac has two significant functions: 1) blood cell formation and 2) the formation of primitive sex cells that will eventually become the sperm and eggs of the developing baby.

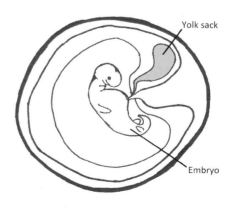

Yolk sack

Embryo

Figure 2.5

In the week after the gonadal ridges appear, these primordial sex cells migrate from the yolk sac and seed into the gonadal ridge, where they multiply copiously, resulting in billions of potential egg or sperm cells. Only now, in response to this seeding, does the gonadal ridge switch on to become either an ovary or a testis, depending upon the nature of the seeding cells.

Ponder this extraordinary phenomenon for a moment! It's the complete inverse of what we'd anticipate. We would expect the ovaries and testes to form first and then 'grow' the egg and sperm populations inside them. Yet the reverse occurs. I wonder why? The sequence says something profound about the primacy of our germinal sex cells. Life puts such store in propagating the species that even before a new individual is formed, the seeds of the succeeding generation are already present. And it's the seeds' presence that switches the organs housing them into ovaries or testes.

This has a unique repercussion for women, who are born with all the eggs they will ever release during their lifetime. What it means is that the tiny egg cell which began 'you' at fertilisation was already present in your mother's ovary, whilst she was growing inside her mother's womb. Symbolically, this is significant and graphically illustrates the tenacity of the mother–daughter connection, as well as the lineage interconnection. Like Russian dolls one inside the other, our own personal maternal DNA was at one point three generational layers deep. This one-inside-the-other-inside-the-other phenomenon is an exclusively female capacity that has no equivalent in father–son relations. Sperm are produced anew all the time and the sperm of a given man was never at any time inside his father, let alone his father's father.

Now that the sex cells have seeded the gonadal ridge, another fascinating qualifier appears. The gonadal ridge will only differentiate into a testis if the critical genetic messenger on the Y chromosome is present. If it's not, then even with a Y chromosome, ovaries will develop. Once again the *female* form is the default setting, which is modified by an additional factor to transform it into maleness.

In its sexually indifferent stage, the embryo is capable of developing into either sex. As we saw earlier, prior to the seeding of the gonads, there's a double duct system and a common external outlet. The two sets of tubes are known respectively as the **Mullerian** ducts (female) and the **Wolffian** ducts (male), named after the embryologists who first discovered them about a century ago.

Why the extravagance of *both* sets of tubes? Why not just one, determined genetically by the XX or XY chromosome combination? We might have simply had a single set of tubes, pre-wired to develop into either female ducts or male ones. Yet, nature opted for both. In females, the Wolffian ducts degenerate, and the Mullerian ducts develop into uterine tubes, uterus, and inner part of the vagina. In males, the Mullerian ducts degenerate and the Wolffian ducts develop into the epididymis, the vas deferens, the seminal vesicle, the prostate and the Cowper's glands. (Figure 2.6)

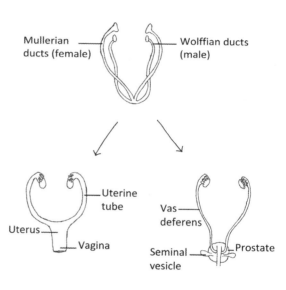

Figure 2.6

The male system will only develop if the embryonic testes are present and secrete the right hormones. Two vital hormones needed for male development are: 1) **testosterone**, which causes the Wolffian ducts to differentiate into the male internal organs and tubes and 2) **Mullerian Inhibiting Hormone (MIH)**, which causes the female ducts to degenerate.

In the female embryo, the female gonads need not necessarily be present for the female organs to develop; apparently they'll develop anyway. However, if for some reason the embryonic testes do not produce testosterone, the genetic male will develop female structures and genitals. As Elaine Marieb describes:

"It appears that the female pattern of reproductive structures has an intrinsic ability to develop and in the absence of testosterone, proceeds to do so, regardless of the embryo's genetic makeup".[4]

This further underscores the default female setting. Similarly, if an embryonic female is exposed to testosterone (for example, if the mother has an androgen-producing tumour) the embryo will have ovaries but will develop male ducts and a penis as well.

2) Differentiation of the genitals

The next phase of sex differentiation is the externalising of femaleness or maleness in the genitals and this part of the process displays the same common denominator we've already seen in the gonads. The external genitals and the vagina develop from identical structures in both sexes, not from the internal tubes but from a small projection of tissue on the pelvic surface called the **genital tubercle.** (Figure 2.7)

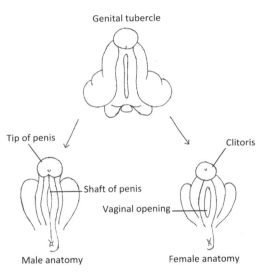

Figure 2.7

During the embryo's sexually indifferent stage, the tubercle has an opening, the **urethral groove**, surrounded by tissues called **urethral folds.** On either side of these folds are the **labio-scrotal swellings.** During week eight of the embryonic phase, the genital structures begin a series of rapid developments. The output of male or female hormones from the now active gonads is what initiates this outer sexual differentiation.

In females, the genital tubercle becomes the **clitoris**, the unfused urethral folds become the **labia minora**, and the unfused labio-scrotal folds become the **labia majora**. The urethral groove continues in females as the **vestibule** of the vulva. In males, the same tissue which became the clitoris grows to form the **penis** (head and erectile bodies), while the urethral folds fuse together to form the **penile urethra**, and the labio-scrotal swellings join in the middle to form the **scrotum**.

From this information, we can see how the genital differentiation process is intrinsically open to endless variations on a theme, with potential for way more diversity than is commonly recognised. For whatever reason, the process modifies in uniquely individual ways, so for intersex people, their genitals are *"organised somewhere between the standard female and standard male configurations".* [5] As Emily Nagoski points out, there's nothing 'wrong' with their genitals, any more than there's anything wrong with having large or small labia: we all have the same parts, just organised differently.

3) Differentiation of the brain

The critical time for full development of the genital tract is about 50–60 days after fertilisation when the embryo is 2–3cm in length and weighs about 1gm. At about the same time and governed by the same hormones, a similar process of sex differentiation appears to occur in the embryonic brain. Whilst all of us, male and female, derive from identical tissues and structures, and share common ground in these early weeks, the dramatic differences that will colour the rest of our lives as female or male are already beginning to occur inside our brains. In 1973, for example, it was shown for the first time that female and male brains have structural differences:

> *"The best example concerns a specific region (now called the sexually dimorphic nucleus) in the anterior region of the hypothalamus that has a distinctive synaptic pattern in each sex."* [6]

Scientists theorised that the brain's organisation into a specifically female or male 'setting' occurs in the embryo around the time of sex differentiation. Just as we saw with the gonads and the genitals, it seems the brain has a basically female template. Intervention in the form of testosterone is needed to alter that template into the male brain pattern. If the embryo is genetically female and no testosterone is present, the basic female pattern remains unchanged.

By contrast, male embryos are exposed to enormous amounts of testosterone (some four times the level experienced in infancy and boyhood!) right at the critical time when their brains are forming. During brain development, there are windows of nerve cell growth influenced by testosterone. Exposure to the right amount of male hormone at this time is crucial because the brain cells acquire a 'set' which is highly resistant to change subsequently.

These findings were deduced by studying individuals for whom the sexing of the brain varied from the male/female dichotomy. For example, a male embryo might produce enough testosterone to develop male sex organs but not enough to masculinise the brain, so he experiences having a 'female' brain in a male body. Similarly, a female embryo exposed to higher than usual amounts of testosterone ends up with a 'male' brain in a female body. Timing is critical. Once the brain is 'set' into its male or female pattern, no amount of exposure to opposite sex hormones will affect it. Dr Irene Elia describes the implications of this phenomenon for female fertility:

> "...the hypothalamus, the crescent of midbrain tissue in direct communication with the pituitary, apparently changes permanently after exposure to fetal androgens. If it receives an early dose of male hormone, it will not be able to cyclically release factors that trigger ovulation. Only the female hypothalamus, **unexposed** in fetal life to androgens, will be able to do this."[7]

What this means is that a female embryo exposed to male hormones won't experience the usual process that governs the menstrual cycle when she reaches the age of puberty or thereafter.

There's enormous controversy about brain-derived sex differences (including this notion of the brain acquiring a 'set'), fuelled partly by fear of gender stereotyping and also by the limitations of our current knowledge. Here's my view. Our lived experience shows us the obvious differences between male and female brains in our ways of thinking, perception, sensing, knowing, communicating, sexual response, spatial awareness, relationship potential and so on. Some differences are culturally constructed, some are by nature. Baby girls, for example, will seek out and maintain eye contact more readily than baby boys. To me, it makes sense that high testosterone levels in a male embryo would significantly alter brain structure and function in ways that affect behaviour. Understanding this difference has made me more respectful of maleness and has stopped me making men 'wrong'.

It's also important to acknowledge that the brain is much more sophisticated than the gonads or genitals because of its connection to consciousness. So while prenatal hormones may predispose an individual to subsequent patterns of behaviour, those behavioural differences can't be attributed solely to biology. As Lesley Rogers cautions:

> ".. it is most unlikely that the brain obeys the same rules of development as the gonads, as the gonads are fairly simple organs, whereas the brain is the most complex organ in the body."[8]

A complex web of genes, hormones, culture, socialisation, history and personal experience all contribute to our sexual differences and the ways in which our brains function. We are not determined by our biology. Our social and cultural contexts, which vary enormously from place to place and are constantly subject to change, play a huge role in behavioural differences.

Gender Diversity

What's so exciting about this embryological sexual differentiation process is the light it sheds on the multiple opportunities during our earliest beginnings for diversity around gender. The presence of *both* primordial duct systems, a common genital tubercle and hormonally mediated changes in the brain provide ample opportunity for endless variations from what is commonly regarded as a mutually exclusive male/female binary. These embryonic processes may comprise the physiological underpinning of the gender revolution now changing the landscape of how we comprehend gender.

Understanding that there's really no such thing as a clear-cut male/female divide is liberating for everyone. In addition to male/female, we now acknowledge intersex people (who can't be easily categorised as female or male), non-binary individuals (who don't identify as male or female), androgynous folk, transgender and gender-fluid people. Knowledge of the sexual differentiation process enables us to appreciate that there are endless individual expressions on a wide-ranging human spectrum that had its origins in a common beginning. To be human is to be unique and the process of becoming gendered is no exception.

What happens to us as embryos has profound consequences for the remainder of our lives. As females this means that we are wired differently from men, or to be more accurate, men are wired differently from us. And since we live in a patriarchal culture with a predominantly masculine psychology, many of the processes, assumptions, attitudes, behaviours and spirituality that are based on male experience may have little relevance or meaning for our distinctly female way of being, which brings its own unique perspective and an altogether different contribution.

Embryo to Fetus

By the end of the embryonic phase at eight weeks, the embryo has blossomed into nearly 1 billion cells with more than 90% of the anatomic structures found in adults. The limbs have formed, along with tiny fingers and toes. The skeleton is complete and the protruding tail has disappeared. The head occupies half the body volume, and eyes, ears, nose and mouth are clearly visible. The tiny embryo is distinctly male or female and has now reached a threshold in its development.

Sex differentiation marks the completion of the embryonic phase and the change in status is accompanied by a new name: **fetus** ('*young in the womb*'). The metamorphosis from sexually undifferentiated embryo into female fetus is a significant milestone in our incarnation of the female body form. From here on, most of the changes involve further tissue and organ specialisation, growth, and changes in body proportion.

During this phase, the fetus grows from 3cm and 1gm to about 36cm and 3kg! At the end of this time, the fully grown baby is ready to make its way into the world through the momentous process of birth. That process leads us now to a closer look at the extraordinary female reproductive system, by which conception, gestation and birthing are made possible. Before we look at the separate organs, we need a context for appreciating the whole organism out of which these amazing organs emerge. That's the subject of the next short chapter.

Reflection

What I now know about becoming female that I didn't know before is…

What I most love and appreciate about becoming female is…

When I reflect on this information, what strikes or moves me is…

Affirmation

I respect and honour my choice to differentiate as female, as I respect other people's choice to differentiate in their own way.

Suggestion

Check out this TED talk by Alexander Tsiaras who takes incredible photos of the human body. These are his stunning pictures of the first moments of human life: https://www.youtube.com/watch?v=fKyljukBE70

Section Two

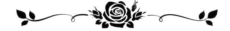

The Female Reproductive System

Chapter Three

The Holographic Template For Health

As we saw in the Introduction, our physical body is the platform from which we, as spiritual beings, experience being human. Our reproductive system is one of the defining characteristics of our gender. As females, we can bear offspring and men cannot. It is deeply meaningful that we're privileged to live the spirituality of our female body processes. Our reproductive organs embody a rich symbolic significance that adds incredible depth to our lives. Delving into these deeper aspects enables a whole new world to open up.

As you learn about and understand how your body processes work, you take more intentional ownership of your femaleness. You begin to appreciate its design and align with it, instead of working to get on top of it, or trying to succeed in spite of it. Even if you have no interest in getting pregnant, are not able to conceive or are past child-bearing, understanding these amazing capacities will deepen your self-respect. Better yet, you'll begin to access the powerful spirituality residing in your body, which is your unique contribution to the world. Most of us have grown up with no awareness of this cosmological potential, so it's very exciting that we are now awakening to it.

Far from being a random act of nature, there's purpose to our female embodiment beyond creating babies. Being female consists of infinitely more than possession of a female reproductive system and the ability to produce young. It has as much to do with our consciousness and the way in which our intellect, emotions, sensitivity, perceptions, intuitions and spirituality inform that consciousness. At the same time, living the relational potential of the female body can generate a potent biological leadership that's critically needed at this time in Earth's evolution.

Before we begin our in-depth study of our female organs, it's important to remember that our reproductive system functions in concert with all our other systems: circulatory, lymphatic, digestive, respiratory, urinary, endocrine, muscular, skeletal and central nervous systems. In Chapter One, we saw how the *organism* is the primary reality. All our systems are governed by our mind (conscious and unconscious), our will and the quest of our spirits. What's more, our entire organism exists as a dynamic flow of energy in relationship with our social and cultural contexts, our Planet and the greater Universe. As Deepak Chopra says, your physical body is not a material object – it is a flow of energy.[1] In fact, energy is our primary reality.

Energy as the Primary Reality

In the Introduction, we saw how the model of the Universe as a machine resulted from an artificial separation of matter and spirit. Thankfully, this worldview began to transform around the turn of the 20th century because the discovery of electro-magnetic fields required new theories to account for the nature of reality.[2] Developing technologies allowed previously invisible energies to be seen and measured for the first time. The scientific revolution that followed described Earth as a living organism and the Universe as a web of energy with wave-like patterns of interconnection. This new science completely inverted previous notions of separate, isolated things by claiming that everything in the Universe is interrelated and interdependent.[3] In the following paragraphs, I include some brushstrokes of the new science, so you can make the shift out of the old paradigm into the new one.

Quantum science redefined the Universe as teeming with probabilities rather than certainties. It is much more unpredictable and mysterious than previously realised and – most radical of all – it is a *participatory* Universe, where the act of observation changes what is observed.[4] The birth of the quantum paradigm opened up new ways of thinking about the nature of reality and gave us a new way of understanding what it means to be human. The body began to be conceptualised as a condensation of energy and scientists discovered that cells vibrate in specific frequencies. Remember the vibrational continuum described in the Introduction, in which we move continually between the world of humanity and the world of divine truth? Our patterns of thinking alter the frequencies in our cells in ways that contribute to dis-ease or wellbeing.[5]

Quantum science has shown us that *energy* is the primary reality out of which matter dynamically unfolds, in fields united by an underlying wholeness. Physicist David Bohm called this underlying wholeness the *implicate order,* a foundational state out of which third dimensional reality becomes manifest as the *explicate order.*[6] Implicate comes from the Latin root meaning '*to enfold*', so the implicate order can be thought of as the creative, dynamic and mysterious underpinning of the Universe, in which everything is enfolded. It could be considered the mind of God or the Divine Womb. Explicate means '*to unfold*', so in the explicate order, things are unfolded, each occupying its own space – not as independently existing units, but as manifestations of the implicate order, birthed into being.

This paradigm shift is important because it means the description of the Universe and the human body as machines is no longer tenable. Instead, Bohm proposed the hologram as a more useful metaphor. A **hologram,** from the Greek holos ('*whole*') and gramma ('*message*') is a transparent 3-D image of light beams encoded with information in such a way that the whole remains present in the part. Brain researcher, Dr Karl Pribram, described the brain's deep structure as holographic, saying that it abstracts from the Universe in a manner which can transcend time and space, and also that our senses are processed holographically throughout our entire system.[7] This holographic quality is evident in our bodies, for example, in the acupressure points on our hands and feet that correspond to different organs inside our bodies.

Our body is a holographic projection of our consciousness which is constantly interacting with and influencing the energy field in which we live and move and have our being. Pause for a moment to consider what this means. It means that in a participatory universe, we literally co-create our own reality, principally through our thoughts. These thoughts, beliefs, intentions and emotions create the energy field for our body. The Universe totally supports us in whatever we choose to believe – good or not so good – because we have freedom of choice. So if we choose to change our beliefs about ourselves (which then changes our energy field), we can modify the energy configuration of our body.

Holographic Template for Health

Within our bodies, I believe we have a *holographic template for health* that acts like the energetic scaffolding upon which our physical organs rest. This template is encoded with all the information needed for health and when our organs are aligned with that template, we enjoy good health; when they're out of alignment, our health is compromised.

Misalignment can be caused by many things, including chronically held emotions and unhelpful thoughts and beliefs which, over time, become more and more solidified in our energy field and eventually become manifested as illness and disease.[8] As luminous beings with freedom of choice, we can realign with the template for health to restore balance and create healing. The following story illustrates the potential of working consciously with this holographic template.

> *Katrina was a participant in one of my workshops, during which I did a guided meditation for a group of women to look inside their pelvic bowls to assess their state of health. During this meditation, Katrina saw the inside of her uterus as dark and full of blocked energy. Several months earlier, she'd experienced a miscarriage and now wanted to conceive again. When she came to see me later for a private session, she told me that during the workshop meditation her uterus felt "contracted and withdrawn". I guided Katrina to visualise the holographic template in her pelvis and to use the power of her intent to shift her uterus back into complete alignment with it. She told me afterwards that her womb was tilted forwards and that she felt something like a 'click' as her womb realigned into position. Not long after this, Katrina conceived again and subsequently gave birth to a healthy baby girl.*

We all have innate healing mechanisms within us; when we cut our finger, it will heal if we care for it. So will broken bones. What if the instructions for this healing come from our holographic template? When we access that template, we can realign whatever is out of alignment.

Like the scientists of old, the textbook model of human anatomy has broken down our wholeness into separate bits like uterus, tubes and ovaries. So as we explore the following chapters, we need to remember that we are, in fact, whole organisms of energy movement. Then the sequential exploration of each organ can enable us to travel through our brilliant inscape, admiring its magnificent views and learning its inspiring secrets. Knowledge is power, so let's now begin at the innermost point of the female reproductive system – the powerhouse ovaries!

Reflection

What I now know about the world and my body that I didn't know before is…

What I most love and appreciate about my body as an energy being is…

When I reflect on this information, what strikes or moves me is…

Affirmation

My body houses a holographic template for perfect health and I align with it perfectly.

Suggestion

Google some energy fields now rendered visible. Some examples are:

1) NASA's visual depiction of the Earth's magnetic field: https://www.nasa.gov/mission_pages/sunearth/news/gallery/Earths-magneticfieldlines-dipole.html

2) The Institute of HeartMath's video on the human heart's electro-magnetic field: https://www.heartmath.org/resources/videos/science-of-the-heart/

Chapter Four

❧～～❧

The Ovaries

Roughly the same size and shape as unshelled almonds, our two **ovaries** are among the most dynamic, creative and potent organs in our body. Measuring about 3cm X 1.5cm X 1cm, they lie well-protected behind the uterus, against the bony lateral pelvic wall, roughly 10–13cm below the waist. Attached to the uterus by the ovarian ligaments, these dynamic little powerhouses are covered with a fibrous capsule quaintly called the **tunica albuginea** ('*white coat*'), which forms a protective outer coat. Beneath this is the **cortex** ('*outer layer*') which houses the follicles and the egg cells. In the middle of the ovary is the **medulla** ('*marrow*' or '*pith*'), which contains blood vessels, nerves, lymph vessels and cells that produce a continuous baseline of oestrogen. (Figure 4.1)

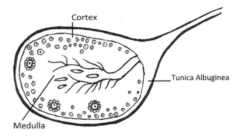

Figure 4.1

The word ovary comes from the Latin **ovarium** meaning '*egg receptacle*'. Whilst they do indeed house the egg cells, they also perform another vital function: production of the female sex hormones, oestrogen and progesterone. These two functions – egg housing and hormone production – are inextricably linked, as we shall see.

The best way to gain an appreciation of the astonishing dynamism of the ovaries is to track the three phases of their monthly cycle. Beginning at menstruation, the **follicular phase** culminates in **ovulation**, which in turn gives way to the **luteal phase** which leads onto the next menstruation.

Let's now look at each of them in turn.

1) THE FOLLICULAR PHASE: (approximately days 1–10)

A remarkable transformation process distinguishes this phase. Within the ovarian cortex, the egg cells are housed in tiny sac-like structures called **follicles** ('*little bags*') measuring about 0.25mm in diameter. Some follicles go through an extraordinary developmental progression as they mature on their way to releasing an egg.

While most of the follicles are immature, at any given time in an adult woman, there are egg cells and follicles at various stages of development because the process is continuous. At the beginning of each cycle, 6 to 12 of the immature or **primordial** follicles begin to grow. At this stage, only one layer of follicle cells surrounds the egg. Under the influence of **follicle stimulating hormone (FSH)** from the pituitary gland in the brain, this surrounding layer deepens to two cells. These cells become **granulosa cells**, which will eventually become the egg's **corona radiata** once it is released. The follicle is now called a **primary follicle**.

During this stage, connective tissue from the ovarian cortex condenses around the outside of the follicle forming the **theca folliculi** ('*box around the follicle*'). Both these layers – the **theca** and the **granulosa** – then collaborate in an ingeniously cooperative fashion to create the hormone oestrogen. Here's how it happens. As the follicle grows, the theca cells begin to produce the more generic sex hormones, **androgens**. The granulosa cells then cleverly absorb and convert the raw androgen into oestrogen. Simultaneously, the granulosa cells also secrete the substance of the **zona pellucida**, which will become the egg's tough leathery transparent shell. When the egg reaches a certain stage of growth, a fluid-filled space begins to surround it. Known as the **antrum** ('*cave*'), this watery cavity continues to expand and is responsible for the remainder of the follicle's growth. The follicle is now described as a **secondary follicle**.

About one week into the ovarian cycle, a mysterious selection process occurs. Of primordial follicles which become **secondary follicles,** only one – the largest or **dominant** one – continues on to ovulation. Once the selection occurs, the remaining follicles simply degenerate. (Figure 4.2)

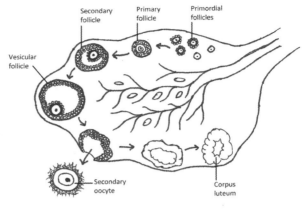

Figure 4.2

2) THE OVULATORY PHASE:
(approximately days 11-14 or when ovulation occurs)

The dominant follicle continues to swell, ballooning out on the surface of the ovary like a blister. Around ovulation, it expands to a massive 1.5cm! When you consider that the ovary itself is only about 3cm long, you get some idea of the scale of this stretch! It is now known as the **vesicular (or Graafian) follicle**.

Fluid-filled spaces begin to appear between the granulosa cells surrounding the egg and the outer follicle cells, freeing the egg and corona radiata from the rest of the follicle. Simultaneously, the egg itself undergoes a rapid change. Hormonal signals initiate the completion of the first meiotic division, which was originally begun and suspended in the embryo many years, even decades, earlier! The egg divides into a **secondary oocyte** and a much smaller **polar body** (which disintegrates), so it retains 23 pairs of chromosomes.

Everything is now ready for the climax of the ovarian cycle: ovulation! In response to a surge of luteinising hormone from the pituitary gland in the brain, the outer wall of the follicle thins, oozing fluid, whilst the muscle-like cells of the theca layer contract powerfully. The result is an impressive rupture of the ovarian surface that propels the egg towards the actualisation of its destiny. Surrounded by its corona radiata, the egg launches itself out into the pelvic cavity still afloat in the antral fluid. Photos capturing this moment reveal the majestic egg hovering amidst swirling fluids and arcs of radiating cells. (Figure 4.3)

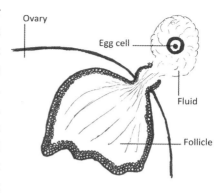

Figure 4.3

Ovulation Pain:

Some women experience this event as ovulation pain. On occasions, the whole pelvis may feel swollen and tender, while at other times, there may be a sharp twinge low down towards the groin, usually on one side of the pelvis. The sensation can last from a couple of hours to a whole day. Between 25 and 50% of women regularly experience some pain before, during or after ovulation. There are a several possible origins. It may be caused by the rapid swelling of the follicle on the ovarian surface just prior to ovulation – hardly surprising considering that *stretch!* It may be due to the spilling of 6–7ml of antral fluid from the ruptured follicle into the pelvis, causing local irritation to the surrounding tissues. Or it may be caused by smooth muscle contraction in the uterine tubes as they prepare for ovulation. No one really knows. A hot water bottle or heat pack on the pelvis helps relieve discomfort and it usually passes within a few hours.

It's believed the ovaries alternate, taking turns to release the egg cell, which seems rather remarkable. How do they remember which one ovulated last? Very occasionally (1–2% of all ovulations), two egg cells mature together and are released within 24hrs of each other. If each is fertilized, the result will be fraternal (non-identical) twins. By contrast, identical twins occur when one single fertilised egg divides in two, producing two genetically identical offspring.

3) THE LUTEAL PHASE: (approximately days 15–28 or menses)

After the rupture of ovulation, what's left of the follicle undergoes a rapid and astonishing transformation. Instead of degenerating as might be expected after such a dramatic event, the remaining theca and granulosa cells in the ruptured follicle organise themselves, almost overnight into another completely different actively secreting gland. This process is known as **luteinisation**. Just think about that for a moment. In any other part of the body, a wound like that would be noticeably painful and need time to heal; imagine a blister that size on your hand or foot, and how long it would take to regrow the surface layer of skin so it was no longer tender and raw. Yet the tissue in the ovaries is so dynamic and creative that the repair is simultaneously a creative act. Here's how it happens.

First, the antrum fills with clotted blood which is gradually resorbed. Then within hours, the remaining granulosa cells enlarge greatly, and newly formed capillaries grow into the centre of the follicle. Once again, granulosa and theca cells cooperate brilliantly. This new gland, called the **corpus luteum** (*'yellow body'*), now begins to secrete the second major female hormone, **progesterone**, as well as some oestrogen. Progesterone is the hormone that prepares for pregnancy (*pro* = for, *gestation* = pregnancy). The intelligence that orchestrates such a rapid healing, transformation and re-creation is truly to be admired.

If the ovulated egg cell is not fertilised and doesn't implant in the womb lining, the corpus luteum reaches it maximum development by about ten days, after which it rapidly degenerates and is **catabolised**, i.e. broken down into simpler molecules. The remaining tissue is then called the **corpus albicans** (*'white body'*) and this continues shrinking until after several months, it is finally removed by scavenging cells called **macrophages** (*'big eaters'*).

If conception does occur, the corpus luteum continues producing progesterone and oestrogen, a hormonal signal that prevents menstruation and promotes the continued growth of the uterine lining. In fact, the corpus luteum persists until the third month of pregnancy, by which stage it has grown as large as 3cm in diameter. This enables time for the placenta to take over the production of oestrogen and progesterone.

At any given time in a woman's ovaries, all stages of follicle growth and development can be seen because the process is continuous. The textbook ovarian cycle is described as 28 days, with ovulation occurring around day 14. However in real life, the normal range of cycle length varies enormously, both from woman to woman and in the same woman, from month to month. When there is a change in cycle length, it occurs in the follicular phase at the beginning of the cycle and is caused by an early or late ovulation. The timing of ovulation can vary from as early as seven days after the beginning of the cycle to as long as 30 or more days after menses.

Many factors can disrupt the finely tuned sequence of hormones governing the ovarian cycle to cause a delay in ovulation: sickness, stress, travel, emotional turbulence and even positive stresses like a wedding or buying a new house. This is because the part of the brain that mediates the release of the hormones responsible for initiating ovulation, the **hypothalamus**, is also the emotional control centre. It's like the brain says, 'Now is not a good time to have a baby' and it waits for more conducive circumstances before resuming the normal release of the fertility hormones. Once ovulation has occurred, however, whether at Day 7 or Day 30, menstruation will follow within 12–16 days, unless the egg is fertilised. This final (luteal) phase of the cycle is a relative constant.

THE EGG (OR OOCYTE):

No chapter on the ovaries would be complete without an in-depth study of the egg cell. Eleven times heavier than the next largest cell in the body, the egg is by far the biggest cell in our body and the most unique in terms of its function. As a spherical ball of cytoplasm, the egg is a solitary creature, an unusual property for cells, which usually congregate together to create tissues. So let's look at the oocyte, both in its individual development (ontogenically), and in its evolutionary aspects.

Oogenesis: (*'egg generation'*)

As we saw in Chapter Two on Sex Differentiation, the sex cells that eventually become a woman's eggs were already present when she was an eight-week-old embryo. The sheer number of these primitive cells is staggering! Life's investment in propagating the species is evident in the extravagance of the five-month-old fetus, where there can be as many as *7 million* primordial sex cells! The number declines to roughly 2 million at birth and continues to decline until at puberty about 500,000 remain. Given that in her entire reproductive lifetime a woman will only ovulate between 400–500 eggs, this is a super-abundance!

Oogenesis (the maturation of the egg cell) takes decades to complete. We saw earlier how the primary oocytes remain 'stalled' in the first phase of cell division (meiosis 1) for years, until they are ovulated from their follicle. Only under the influence of the **luteinising hormone** surge that triggers ovulation, does the primary oocyte complete meiosis 1 and enter meiosis 2, becoming a **secondary oocyte**. It then stalls again and will complete meiosis 2 only if a sperm actually penetrates its membranes. After this, it is technically known as an **ovum**. If the oocyte is not fertilised, it degenerates within 24hrs.

Difference Between Female and Male Sex Cells

There are striking differences between female and male sex cells. The oocyte is just visible with the naked eye, measuring roughly 0.14mm in diameter, which is about the size of a full-stop. In size, it is equivalent to about 60,000 sperm. Only 400–500 eggs are ovulated by any given woman, while sperm are produced in the same quantities every half a second. Oocytes can wait decades to be released and survive only 24hrs. Sperm production is continuous and sperm can survive in optimum conditions for five days or more.

Whilst the oocyte has evolved in favour of substance, the sperm has divested substance in exchange for mobility. The two cooperate beautifully together. Human evolution has seen the development of a large, slow-moving egg with substantial cytoplasm, and much smaller sperm with almost no cytoplasm and the ability to seek out their mate. The unique advantages of both sex cells, diverging so much in size, shape and behaviour, contribute to the success of fertilisation. As individual cells, they are at the end of the rope; yet when they fuse, new life becomes possible.

Unique Qualities of the Egg:

In her book *The Female Animal*, Dr Irene Elia ventures an interesting observation of the egg cell:

> *"In their twin capacities to engulf and nurture genetic material from sperms, eggs are unique. No cells except eggs incorporate and support the genetic material of other cells."* [1]

In its capacity to incorporate another cell, the ovum enacts at a microscopic level what a woman does in pregnancy. The ovum's action at fertilisation prefigures the larger body process. As we saw in Chapter One, the egg's boundary penetration allows the intimate fusion of both sets of genetic material. At the cellular level, the egg displays an active receptivity, incorporation and relational quality. As Elia elaborates further:

> *"Lack of motility (the cell's ability to move itself across relatively long distances) in eggs must not be equated with lack of activity. Eggs are very active. After taking in the tiny sperm, they supply energy and genetic data for embryonic development, and may also repair chromosome damage in sperm-cell genes."* [2]

Apparently the egg cytoplasm contains a special kind of ribonucleic acid called **mRNA** (messenger RNA) which can initiate the first stages of development after fertilisation, without receiving directives from the nuclear chromosomes. Normally these mRNA are dormant and only become activated after fertilisation when they become what Elia calls *"the template for the first ten to twenty hours of embryonic life"*.

The egg makes another vital contribution to the development of the embryo through tiny organelles known as mitochondria. As we saw earlier, mitochondria are power capsules that move around and change shape constantly inside our cells. Mitochondria contain their own genetic material and it's now widely believed that they were originally a form of bacteria that colonised our cells and learned to live within them symbiotically.

Whenever a cell has high energy requirements, lots of mitochondria are present. As you might imagine, the ovum is richly supplied with them, reflecting its dynamic nature. The DNA inside the mitochondria of our egg cell is a secondary source of maternal DNA, as Joan Borysenko observed: *"The ovum also contributes genetic material to the offspring above and beyond what is present in nuclear chromosomes."*[3] This mitochondrial DNA helps to direct nuclear genes and thus actively contributes to the development of the embryo. This secondary DNA also has some very interesting evolutionary properties, as Borysenko explains:

> *"The mitochondrial DNA in our cells today is very similar to what it was at the dawn of creation since it has not been contaminated by the messy genetic mixing that occurs when males and females pool their genes – since the sperm's mitochondria are lost when the egg incorporates the sperm. So in tracing the origins of mitochondrial DNA, biologists have also been able to trace our matrilineal family tree back to an African Eve, sometimes called Mitochondrial Eve, who lived somewhere between 150,000 and a quarter of a million years ago."*[4]

Who would have guessed that such a story of antiquity and preservation is hidden away inside the power capsules of our ovum?

These active, intelligent properties are the perfect embodiment of Elia's contention that both females and eggs could be said to 'egg on' life:

> *"...the verb "to egg" offers a number of appropriate although linguistically accidental meanings that might be applied to females and their sex cells. "To egg" meaning "to goad" or "to incite to action" is often a female property. Her presence or the presence of her eggs may attract males, instigate competition among them and provoke spawning or copulation."*[5]

Although Elia is talking about female animals in general, as humans we belong to that class of animals called mammals. So eggs are something we share not only with other mammals, but with females of all other classes.

Through evolution, land vertebrates tried out *"leathery shells, hard shells, earth nests, and twig nests, and finally internalized the nests, moistening, protecting and feeding embryos within their own bodies."*[6] As human females, our eggs evolved the tough 'shell' of the zona pellucida, which although it looks soft, is nonetheless quite sturdy and difficult to break. For some women, toughness of the zona can cause fertility problems because the sperm can't break through to fertilise the egg. In reproductive technology, the procedure called **ICSI** (intra cytoplasmic sperm injection) manually penetrates the zona with a very fine instrument, injecting the sperm right into the oocyte to trigger fertilisation, a procedure known to have good results.

Symbolic Significance of the Egg:

The magnificent ovum is without doubt, an exceptional dimension of our female heritage. Our eggs are supreme nurturers of life. They actively house and protect our genetic treasure. Uniquely in cell-land, they incorporate sperm and provide the substance and instructions for the first hours of new human life. They heal, repair and sustain, and they are bursting with creative energy. Our eggs are our seed. A seed is germinal, holding within itself the keys to its own actualisation. It is the source of what it to come. And as source, it possesses spiritual power. We will return to this image of the seed shortly.

Back to the Ovaries:

The ovaries are truly remarkable in their function and behaviour. As we've seen, they produce the female hormones that make a woman look and feel like a woman – particularly oestrogen, which affects skin, bones, muscles, mucus membranes, uterus, tubes, vagina, vulva, breasts and brain. Oestrogen also produces the secondary sex characteristics, which begin the transformation of a girl into a young woman at puberty:

enlargement of breasts, growth of pubic hair, broadening of the hips and rounded appearance.

Far from being inert, passive little structures that simply pump out chemicals, the ovaries are incredibly dynamic and creative. They bring about significant rupture of their surface and then within hours, convert that rupture into an actively secreting endocrine gland. This boundary-breaking of the ovarian surface is part of its healthy design. As Sheila Kitzinger noted:

> *"The extraordinary thing is that though the ovum bursts out of the ovary through a swelling 1.5cm across (roughly the size of a hazelnut), no wound is produced, no scar is left by ovulation, and it happens again and again and again, without causing injury."*[7]

What's more, the ovaries are surprisingly mobile and collaborative. Apparently when the egg's about to rupture from its follicle, the ovary turns its ovulating side towards the open end of the uterine tube to maximise the tube's ability to capture the floating egg. How does it know to do this? It's the same intelligence that's evident throughout the entire female system.

Light of Life:

In her book *Women Who Run With The Wolves,* Clarissa Pinkola Estés writes:

> *"To have the seed means to have the key to life... In Mexico, women are said to carry "luz de la vida", the light of life. This light is located, not in a woman's heart, nor behind her eyes, but 'en los ovarios', in her ovaries."*[8]

We saw earlier how the ovaries perform two functions: egg housing and hormone production, and how the process of releasing the egg from its 'house' is what generates the hormones. Hormones are powerful, consciousness-altering substances which I believe mediate the spirituality in our bodies. They act globally, activating receptors in hundreds of different areas inside our bodies, which is where our consciousness resides. This may be the physiology behind Estés' contention that the light is located in our ovaries.

An example that illustrates this well is the experience of many women taking the Pill. The combined oral contraceptive pill suppresses ovulation, as well as thickening cervical mucus and altering the lining of the uterus. Many women have told me they felt 'terrible' while taking the Pill: depressed, moody, no libido and 'not myself'. For these women, it feels like the light has gone out. When they stop taking the Pill, their light turns on again. This can also occur with hormonal contraceptives like the mini-pill, Mirena, Implanon and Depo Provera, though the return of the light and fertility after Depo can often take months because it has longer-acting chemicals.

Our ovaries are deeply spiritual organs. Through them we access the transpersonal. They connect us with the primordial longing to pass on our genetic lineage to our offspring, to perpetuate down the line. They also embody the abundance, richness and extravagance of life. Our ovaries house our seed and are thus the seat of our fertility. Since always, fertility has inspired in human beings feelings of awe, devotion and an appreciation of the sacredness of the female body. From sources as diverse as archaeology, linguistics, comparative religions and historical records, we know that our earliest ancestors worshipped a female deity, the Goddess, who was revered for Her fertility, abundance and embodiment in Nature. Our fertility touches deep into the meaning of what it is to be human. This is why fertility problems affect us so profoundly. To be human is to create, physically and biologically, spiritually and energetically.

This being the case, and mindful of the manner in which our eggs have evolved, Irene Elia's next comment gives us pause for thought:

> *"...when we manipulate the egg by freezing, enucleating, artificially fertilizing or shutting off its normal cyclic production with contraceptives, we touch the source and possibly change the course of evolution."* [9]

This statement is worth pondering. Remember, the cells that go on to become our ova are amongst the earliest migrations of cells in the embryo. They 'seed' the gonad, switching it on to become an ovary. When we request a prescription for the Pill or enlist reproductive technologies, our focus is on the immediate goal. Yet it's conceivable that these decisions we make as individuals could have repercussions further down the evolutionary path – something worth bearing in mind.

Our eggs and ovaries are our sacred stock, living symbols of mysteries far beyond the capacity of human reason. Never before have we been able to manipulate this sacred territory and directly intervene with the luminous substance of our seed. Had we lived in the ancient times of the Goddess, we would have known what it was to revere the life-giving powers of our fertility, even if we didn't know the precise mechanisms.

Our scientific capacity, with its amazing reproductive technologies, has enabled us to create new human life when it wouldn't otherwise be possible. IVF babies are treasured miracles for their parents, who have often waited years and gone to extraordinary lengths to conceive. Yet the perfunctory use of those technologies, when our seeds are treated like inanimate objects, has the capacity to divest human beings of their spirituality. A baby conceived *in vitro* is not just the sum of its parts, like flour and eggs tossed into a bowl to make a cake. When spirit joins matter we have life; there will always be an element of the sacred at this moment.

At the same time, science has provided us with the technological window that enables us to see the stunningly beautiful ecosystem previously hidden inside our bodies. One only has to look at an electron-microscope photo of an oocyte or fertilised egg to appreciate this gift.

Reflection

What I now know about my ovaries that I didn't know before is…

What I most love and appreciate about my ovaries is…

When I reflect on this information, what strikes or moves me is…

Affirmation

I love my beautiful ovaries! They are full of radiant light and I honour their creativity.

Suggestion

Cup your hands gently on either side of your pelvis with your thumbs at your navel. Your pinky fingers will be about where your ovaries are located. Now breathe six deep breaths down into your pelvis and bring your awareness to your ovaries. Feel their subtle, potent energy. Send them your love and gratitude, thank them for all they do.

Chapter Five

The Oviducts Or Uterine Tubes

The **oviducts** or **uterine tubes** are better known in medical terminology as the **Fallopian tubes**, after the Italian anatomist Gabriello Fallopio (1523–62), who first described them. As the 'arms' of our reproductive system, the tubes are wonderfully active and expressive, as they dance their way through the cycle. Measuring roughly 10cm long and 7mm wide, they stretch up and back from each side of the top of the uterus. For clarity's sake, diagrams usually depict the ovaries and tubes laid out above and beside the uterus. However, *in situ*, they wrap behind the womb and lie well protected in a small pool of abdominal fluid.

The tubes are really extensions of the uterus and are divided anatomically into three main subdivisions: the isthmus, the ampulla and the infundibulum. Let's now look at them in detail. The **isthmus** (*'narrow passage'*) is the tube's narrowest end where it opens into the uterine cavity. While textbook drawings usually portray the tubes as wide, hose-like hollows, in reality their opening into the womb is extremely narrow, measuring **0.5–1mm** in diameter – roughly *the thickness of a strand of cotton!* Given this narrowness, it's easy to understand how the tubes can get blocked with mucus or slight kinks.

As the tube arches up and behind the uterus, the isthmus widens to about 2.5 mm and expands into the **ampulla** (*'flask'*), the midsection which comprises two-thirds of the tube's length. The ampulla, which is about 6 mm in diameter, expands even more into the **infundibulum** (*'funnel'*), which is the 'hand' part of the 'arm'. This open, trumpet-shaped end has about 25 feathery, finger-like projections, known as **fimbriae** (*'fringe'*), which hover over the surface of the ovary like a canopy. With amazing dexterity and care, the fimbriae reach down and actually massage the ovary surface around the time of ovulation, contributing to the follicle's rupture process and possibly soothing the sensations produced by the bulging follicle. (Figure 5.1)

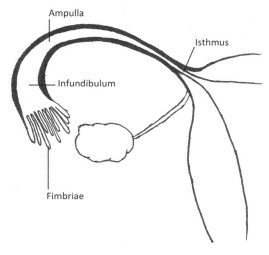

Figure 5.1

The tubes have the extremely important role of providing a safe space for fertilisation to occur. This role involves four functions: 1) transporting sperm towards the egg, 2) capturing the ovulated egg from the ovary surface, 3) creating the perfect environment for the union of sperm and egg, and 4) then transporting the fertilised egg back to the uterus. Far from hanging there like passive appendages, the tubes play a very active role in all of these tasks and are supreme mediators, as we shall see.

Held in place by the broad ligament, the **mesosalpinx** ('*mesentery of the trumpet*'), the tubes are supplied with blood from the ovarian arteries. Structurally, the tube walls are comprised of an inner circular layer and an outer longitudinal layer of smooth muscle. This structure enables them to generate waves of **peristalsis** (just like food going down the oesophagus) and this design helps to actively propel their contents in the right direction.

The lining inside the tube is a highly folded mucus membrane, made up of two different kinds of cells: 1) **ciliated columnar epithelium**, alternating with 2) goblet-shaped **mucosa** cells. (Figure 5.2) The **cilia** (*'eyelash'*) on the epithelial cells are tiny hair-like projections, whose beating

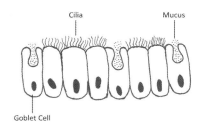

Figure 5.2

creates currents in the tubular fluids that propel sperm and egg along their way. By contrast, the mucosa cells, as their goblet shape suggests, secrete substances that nourish both egg and sperm. During the menstrual cycle, the height of these mucus membrane cells changes so that around ovulation they stretch to about twice their normal size!

Now that we know what they're made of, we can better understand how the oviducts perform their various tasks and how they change their actions throughout the menstrual cycle with incredible flexibility and intelligence. Their most important function is to provide a safe, secure place for fertilisation, which normally occurs in the ampulla, rather than the wide open infundibulum.

An Underwater Garden

Under high-powered magnification, the tube canal resembles a very beautiful underwater coral garden, with fronds waving in the fluid secretions. (See colour plates at the centre of the book.) These images reveal how our body is a sensitive ecosystem, similar to the ecosystem in a coral reef. In her book *Beginning Life*, Geraldine Lux Flanagan captures this scenario eloquently:

> *"Indeed, under great magnification the scene within the channel of the Fallopian tube looks like an underwater ocean landscape. This is a sort of sea within the mother, provided through evolution. It cushions the developing cells, keeps them from dehydration, maintains an even temperature, provides salts and sugars as slight nourishment that the cells absorb, and also contains substances that prepare the cluster for its nesting. At the same time, the fluids lend the transport needed to convey the cluster to its nesting site."* [1]

The tubal liquid, which is quite watery and clear, increases abundantly around ovulation. In such a narrow space, the quality of this fluid is paramount. Clean, clear fluid is essential to effectively transport sperm and fertilised egg. Just like a coral reef, this liquid medium can be contaminated by what's coming into your body. Common contaminants include pesticides and artificial hormones in the food chain, environmental toxins, household cleaning products and allergenic foods. Dairy, for example, is a common allergen that stimulates excess mucus in those sensitive to it, as does wheat. So if eating these foods causes a blocked nose and a tickle at the back of your throat, the fluid inside your tubes will most likely be similarly affected with mucus, which could easily compromise your fertility.

If you think of your body as a sensitive ecosystem rather than a machine, you'll be much more conscious of everything that comes into your body and its potential impacts on your health and fertility. Drinking lots of pure water helps clean the ecosystem and flush out toxins.

Dance of the Uterine Arms

If no egg is waiting in the outer third of the tube, the sperm that succeeded in making it that far cling to the mucosal walls and are nourished while they wait. In the meantime, the tubes are geared up in quite a remarkable way to accomplish their most athletic task: capturing the egg as it bursts from the ovary – which they do with style and panache!

As oestrogen levels rise in the lead-up to ovulation, the tube hovering over the ovulating ovary begins to arch up and position itself in readiness. It reminds me of a cat waiting to pounce! The finger-like fimbriae, which prior to ovulation are docile and inactive, now become erect and begin actively sweeping the ovary surface. Niels Lauersen and Colette Bouchez describe this process well:

> *"Using a gentle sucking action that gently coaxes your egg from its shell, your fimbriae actually reach down and massage your ovary just prior to ovulation. As your egg bursts through your ovary, the fimbriae act like a fertility safety net, catching and gently guiding it inside your fallopian tube."* [2]

Pause and reflect on this action for a moment. I find it very beautiful that the tube is so careful, solicitous and gentle in its treatment of our sacred seed. As the egg bursts forth at ovulation, the beating cilia on the fimbriae create currents in the surrounding fluid, which siphon the egg into the tube, a process that works successfully most of the time. So much dexterity, flexibility and tender care!

Intelligent Agency

As you can see, each month around ovulation, the oviducts dance with extraordinary coordination, mobility and flexibility, which usually goes unnoticed, yet is full of agency. The following true story brilliantly illustrates the tube's enterprising adaptability.

> *Samantha was 38 when her right ovary was removed because of a large ovarian cyst. At the same time, her left uterine tube was also removed because of a thrombosis. Samantha and her husband already had 3 girls and had planned four more children because they really wanted a big family. After the surgery, they were devastated when the gynaecologist informed them that no future pregnancy was possible. However, to their great delight, Samantha's first son was born about a year later. The couple was overjoyed! A miscarriage occurred the following year, followed by the birth of two more sons in quick succession. Samantha then subsequently experienced 3 more early miscarriages.*

With only her *left* ovary and her *right* tube remaining, Samantha had gone on to conceive *seven more times*! This story shows how her right tube was sufficiently flexible and enterprising to seek out the remaining ovary on the opposite side of the pelvis, and successfully capture at least 7 more eggs! When I first heard this story in my early days as a fertility educator, I was filled with admiration and respect. It taught me to never underestimate the intelligence and regenerative capabilities of the female body and to take any medical pronouncements with a grain of salt.

The pre-eminent role of the tubes is to provide the all-important site for fertilisation – the place where spirit ignites matter and where the very beginning of life finds a safe haven. This is the reason behind the tube's concentrated activity around the time of ovulation. In Chapter One, we saw how the fertilised egg takes up to a week to travel down the tube before it reaches a sufficient maturity to be ready to implant in the womb lining.

To ensure our regal sphere travels in the right direction, the beating cilia lining the tube and the peristaltic wave now completely *reverse* their direction from when the sperm were transported up to meet the egg. I find this astonishing! What guides the tube to do this? Whilst it's thought to occur in response to the change in maternal hormones, this reversal seems more deliberate and intentional than simple chemistry. What's more, the swirling current inside the tube is vital to keep the egg moving so as to avoid an untimely implantation inside the tube (an ectopic pregnancy).

Despite their astonishing flexibility and dynamism, the tubes are simultaneously fragile, susceptible organs. Their internal structures – the mucosal folds and hair-like cilia – are easily damaged, and the delicacy of the tissues doesn't lend itself to easy repair. This is why a reversal of tubal ligation (sterilisation) tends to have poor success.

As we've see, the tube's narrow entry into the uterus means it can easily become blocked. In addition to mucus, blocking can be caused by infection after miscarriage, termination of pregnancy or childbirth. A ruptured appendix, peritonitis or pelvic inflammation from sexually transmitted diseases can also create blocks in the tube, as can adhesions from other pelvic diseases or injuries. And a tube can be blocked by muscular spasm or kinking. In fact, blocking and scarring of the tubes is one of the major causes of female subfertility. A technique called **tubal catheterisation,** using x-rays, guide wires and catheters, has been shown to successfully unblock the tubes with minimal damage to their delicate interior. The pregnancy rate following this procedure is as high as 60%,as long as the unblocked tubes are normal and there's no tubal disease. [3]

Ectopic Pregnancy

Occasionally, the fertilised egg doesn't make it into the uterus and implants inside the tube. This is known as an **ectopic** (ecto = *outside*) pregnancy. If the implanting blastocyst continues to develop, the tube could stretch very painfully and rupture, or the blastocyst could be pushed out of the open end of the tube into the pelvis. Either of these outcomes is dangerous and can cause severe internal bleeding, pain and shock. Ectopic pregnancy is potentially life-threatening if not diagnosed and treated promptly, so it's vital to get medical attention immediately if the following symptoms are present and there's any possibility of pregnancy.

Symptoms of ectopic pregnancy include abdominal pain (often one-sided), light vaginal bleeding and faintness. The pain can be sharp and localised, or more generalised. Sometimes there's referred pain in the shoulders because blood loss from an ectopic pregnancy can irritate the lining under the diaphragm at the top of the abdomen. Often the pain is 'colicky', coming and going. If treated early enough, the tube can be flushed out and preserved, though the embryo will be lost. If the pregnancy is more advanced, the tube will either need to be carefully opened surgically and the embryo removed, or else the tube itself removed. Sometimes the embryo will die spontaneously, in which case it may be possible to allow things to resolve naturally, as long as there is close monitoring of the situation.

A number of risk factors increase the likelihood of ectopic pregnancy, particularly smoking. A French study reported that smoking accounted for 35% of the risk associated with ectopic pregnancy.[4] Women smoking over 20 cigarettes a day are four times more vulnerable to an ectopic pregnancy than non-smokers. Previous history of miscarriage, termination, ectopic pregnancy or tubal surgery puts you at greater risk, as does a history of pelvic inflammatory disease, sexually transmitted infection and use of an IUD (intrauterine contraceptive device). Women with damaged tubes, previous fertility problems and those using assisted reproductive technologies are also more at risk.

Paradox of the Uterine Tubes

The oviducts embody a contradictory range of qualities that gives us food for thought. They are soft and pliable, with delicate tissues that are easily damaged, and they are vulnerable to loss and infection. At the same time, they perform a complex series of movements each month. They beat their cilia, create peristaltic waves in both directions, arch and move about in response to the ovary, massage the ripe follicle, and wave their finger-like fronds vigorously enough to create currents that sweep the released egg towards them to be captured. As we've seen, they are amazingly alert, adaptable, sensitive, cooperative and clearly capable of initiative. They are simultaneously sturdy and frail.

An Open System

One intriguing characteristic of the oviducts is that *they're not directly attached to the ovaries and instead, open into the pelvis.* Just as the male tubes, the **vas deferens**, are directly attached to the testes in a closed system, the tubes could have been directly attached at their open ends to the ovaries, thereby ensuring that no eggs would be lost. Instead, the tube's design renders them open and therefore susceptible to loss. Not all ovulated eggs are captured by the waiting tubes; a proportion falls into the pelvis and disintegrates. Despite the vulnerability to loss, however, the process is also remarkably efficient. Eggs *do* make it into the tube to meet with their waiting partners almost all the time!

Symbolism of the Tubes

In their openness, the tubes prefigure some very typical female experiences – familiarity with loss and vulnerability to contamination – both of which are related to that other archetypal experience: boundary penetration. Just as we sometimes 'lose' our egg cells into our pelvis, so we also know the devastating loss of our babies in miscarriage, stillbirth or neonatal death. Some women, like Samantha mentioned earlier, experience multiple losses, which may have a cumulative effect.

The loss of a baby during pregnancy can be a traumatic, even a catastrophic event. When new life quickens inside our body and then dies, we feel it in our deepest self. Death penetrates us to our core, just as our baby's presence once did. The boundary penetration admits both the excitement and beauty of new life, and also the desolation and emptiness of its passing. Navigating the labyrinth of grief and loss is part of being female. As the off-spring bearing sex, we get pregnant, we miscarry, we experience loss. It comes with the territory and teaches us about our resilience and strength. When we avoid pathologising our grief, we learn self-care and compassion.

Even when a pregnancy goes full term with a beautiful baby at the end, we still know the feeling of loss that comes from having been filled for months and then suddenly being empty after the birth. We know the loss of weaning our babies after months of breastfeeding, the loss of their toddlerhood reliance on us as they grow into greater independence, the loss when they go to child-care or school, and on it goes. Being female makes us familiar with loss as an inevitable part of our daily lives.

The experience of boundary penetration also renders us, like the tube, vulnerable to contamination. This is true both literally, as well as symbolically. The tube's openness risks the potential spread of disease or infection from other parts of the reproductive tract into the pelvis and vice versa. Conditions like endometriosis, where tissue from the womb lining migrates out through the tubes into the pelvis, or like pelvic inflammatory disease, where infections from other parts of our bodies find their way in through the tubes, illustrate this kind of vulnerability. Our anatomical openness also renders us susceptible to other contaminants, for example, other people's energy, agendas and emotions. This is particularly the case with our sexual experiences and our birthing, during which we're at our most open and vulnerable.

Nature could have designed the tubes differently. They could have been a closed system and yet they're not. Openness and vulnerability are part of their nature and as a result, the tubes embody characteristics that would not have been needed otherwise. They've developed incredible flexibility and adaptability, and a delicate, dance-like coordination that displays ingenuity, timing, anticipation and teamwork with the ovary.

Symbolically, as the 'arms' and 'hands' of our reproductive system, the tubes reach out to capture and embrace new life in a beautiful gesture of open receptivity. Heedless of risk and loss, they do all in their power to foster the union of egg and sperm. They actively support, protect, nourish and transport the new organism, and most of the time, deliver it safely to its nesting site. As mediators between ovaries and womb, they unassumingly dance their way through each menstrual cycle, going about their tasks with quiet dedication.

Reflection

What I now know about my uterine tubes that I didn't know before is…

What I most love and appreciate about my tubes is…

When I reflect on this information, what strikes or moves me is…

Affirmation

I love the open flexibility of my tubes; they lovingly reach out to embrace new life.

Suggestion

Go out somewhere in Nature and stand amongst some big trees. Stretch out your arms to the sky, like your tubes stretch out from your womb towards your ovaries, and declare out loud: I am open to all the goodness in Life and I give thanks for my beautiful female body!

Chapter Six

The Uterus

The **uterus** (Latin '*womb*') is the preeminent organ that captures, incarnates and expresses the spirit of femaleness. As the offspring-bearing sex, we bear those offspring within our wombs. To me, the uterus is the human expression of the fecundity and sacredness of Earth, whose womb is the molten magma core. Our womb is one of the most sacred, fiery and creative places in our bodies. Before we explore this creative power, let's look at the anatomy of this amazing organ.

The uterus nestles deep in the pelvis between the bladder at the front and the rectum at the back. When we're not pregnant, it's roughly the same size and shape as a small inverted pear, measuring about 7.5cm long by 5cm wide by 2.5cm thick, and weighing about 60gms. Amazingly, by the end of pregnancy, it expands *100 times*, approaching the size of a large watermelon, roughly 28cm long by 24cm wide by 21cm thick, and weighing over 1kg! The magnitude of this expansion speaks of the largesse of spirit surrounding the capabilities of this exceptional organ.

Anatomically the uterus is divided into a number of subdivisions: (Figure 6.1)

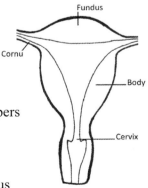

- the **fundus** ('*bottom*') is the end furthest from its opening in the cervix, so although fundus means bottom, it's actually the top of the uterus

- the **cornu** ('*horn*') are the corners where it tapers towards the opening of the oviducts or tubes

- the **body** is the main part of the uterus

- the **cervix** ('*neck*') is the open end of the uterus which extends into the top of the vagina

Figure 6.1

Through the middle of the cervix runs the **endo-cervical canal,** a narrow opening about 6mm wide, which connects the cervix and vagina to the inside of the uterus, known as the **lumen** (*'aperture'*). The vaginal end of the canal, which is doughnut-shaped and can be felt at the top of the vagina, is called the **external os** (*'mouth'*) and the uterine end of the canal, buried deep inside the uterus, is the **internal os**.

Although textbook diagrams depict the inside of the uterus as a balloon-type cavity with lots of empty space, the lumen is actually a narrow, slit-like opening, with the inner walls of the uterus almost touching each other. In its non-pregnant state, it's more accurately a potential space, rather than an open receptacle. In its structural design, the uterus is as complex and paradoxical, as it is sophisticated and elegant. Exploring it is like diving down a rabbit hole; the deeper we go, the more there is to discover. Prepare to be amazed! Its capabilities will astound you.

Structure of the Uterus

The uterine wall is composed of two layers: the **myometrium** and the **endometrium**, each of which is also comprised of several layers. Let's now explore them in detail.

1. The **myometrium** (*'muscle of the uterus'*) is the thick muscular wall comprising the bulk of the uterus; it has three distinct layers: (Figure 6.2)

   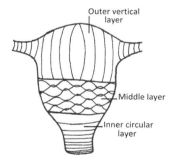

   Figure 6.2

   i) an **outer layer of smooth muscles** running vertically up and down the uterus; these are the muscles that respond to oxytocin and shorten during labour

   ii) a **middle layer of interlacing muscles** and blood vessels that criss-cross the uterine body

   iii) an **inner layer of circular connective tissue fibres** which wrap around the uterus and are most concentrated in the cervix; these fibres thin and open during labour

The outer vertical muscles and the inner circular ones engage in a dance together during labour. As the vertical muscles shorten (or contract), this draws the circular muscles in the cervix open (dilation) and creates thickness in the fundus, so it has the bulk and strength to push the baby down the birth canal. As you can imagine, this shape-shifting in labour is a huge transformation in the structure of the uterus.

2. The **endometrium** (*'within the uterus'*) is the lining of the uterine cavity and it's also made up of two layers: (Figure 6.3)

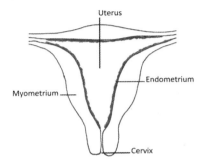

Figure 6.3

i) the **stratum functionalis** (*'functional layer'*), which responds to the ovarian hormones and is shed during menstruation

ii) the **stratum basalis** (*'base layer'*), the thin base layer of cells, which doesn't respond to ovarian hormones and is the source of a new functional layer after each menstruation

In Chapter Nine on menstruation, we explore the fascinating physiology of these two layers of the endometrium much more deeply.

Mobility and Sensitivity of the Uterus

We tend to think of the uterus as a passive organ which, apart from shedding a layer during menstruation, doesn't really do very much until pregnancy. Not so! Like the tubes, the uterus is both energetic and highly mobile. Its position changes continually as the bladder and rectum fill and empty, as the menstrual cycle progresses and in response to other stimuli, especially sexual arousal. As Sheila Kitzinger notes:

> *"The uterus is not just a bag hanging there, but a living network of muscle fibres which, though not under our conscious control, tightens and releases regularly in response to certain stimuli and at special times within the menstrual cycle."* [1]

The womb is also an intelligent and exquisitely sensitive organ, with a tendency to retreat when touched. I'm always mindful of this when speaking with women who've undergone procedures like caesarean surgery, a dilation and curette or IVF. I wonder how their uterus felt when the surgeon was making incisions or touching it with cold instruments. The feminist book, *A New View of a Woman's Body,* describes the dynamic responsiveness of the uterus:

> *"Far from passive, the muscular structure of the uterus contracts in response to sexual stimulation and at the moment of orgasm, and in response to menstruation and breast-feeding, dilation of the cervix or manual stimulation."*[2]

Part of what gives the uterus its mobility is the extensive support network of ligaments, which anchor it securely in the pelvis, allowing for expansive growth during pregnancy and the powerful contractions of labour. Providing the main support are the **transverse cervical ligaments**, which run sideways from the cervix and top of the vagina to the side walls of the pelvis. The **utero-sacral ligaments** extend from the cervix, encircling the rectum and attaching to the front of the sacrum, while the **pubo-cervical ligament** runs from the cervix, underneath the bladder and attaches to the pubic bone.

Lastly, the **round ligaments** extend from the fundus down the front of the pelvis and over the top of the pubic bone, anchoring in the tissues encircling the vagina. This anchor-point provides a direct connection between the uterus and the vulva. During sexual arousal, the round ligaments shorten, lifting the womb forward and up, at the same time pulling pleasurably on the vaginal sphincter muscle. As well as feeling good, this movement of the uterus is an ingenious design to expand the top of the vagina and move the cervix out of the line of direct impact during lovemaking.

From this extensive ligament network, we can see that the uterus is superbly designed to bear weight, to expand during and retract after pregnancy, to adjust to the increasing pressures and space taken up by a baby *in utero*, and to accommodate the astonishing power of the uterine contractions during labour and birth. Given that three of the four ligaments extend out from the cervix, we can see that the cervix must be an exceptionally strong part of the uterus.

The Uterine Cycle

Like the ovaries, the uterus has its own cycle which is divided into three phases:

1. the **menstrual phase** – the days of bleeding during which the functional layer of the endometrium is shed

2. the **proliferative phase** – the days before ovulation when the functional layer of the endometrium grows back again

3. the **secretory phase** – the days after ovulation when the endometrium prepares for possible implantation of an embryo

In Chapter Nine, we explore these three phases of the uterine cycle in great detail. Menstruation is such a significant part of being female that I've devoted an entire chapter to this extraordinary process. Most women in Western culture have no idea of the spiritual potential of their bleeding and the potent resource available to us when we're receptive to it. The entire menstrual cycle is orchestrated by the release of hormones from the pituitary gland, in dialogue with the ovaries, through sophisticated hormonal feedback systems. Female hormones are such a huge topic that I've added my e-book, *Female Hormones,* as a bonus with this book, freely available from the website www.ActivateYourFemalePower.com.

THE CERVIX

The **cervix** (*'neck'*) is such a remarkable part of the uterus, with its own unique structure, characteristics and functions, that it almost deserves to be respected as a separate organ in its own right. As the portal into the uterus, it allows sperm to enter and as we shall see, actively encourages them around the time of ovulation by producing **cervical mucus**. During childbirth, the cervix undergoes an extraordinary stretch in which its opening dilates from 6mm to a whopping 10cm to release the baby from the womb.

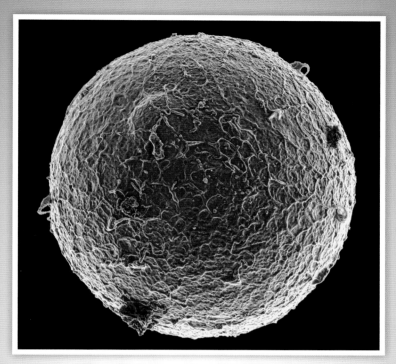

1. Egg cell and sperm

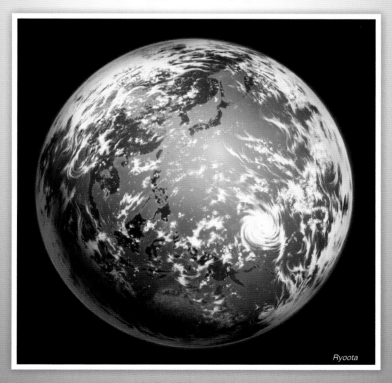

Ryoota

2. Earth from space

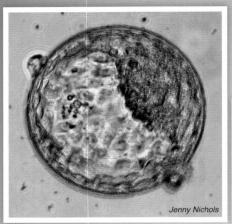

Jenny Nichols

3. Blastocyst with zona pellucida

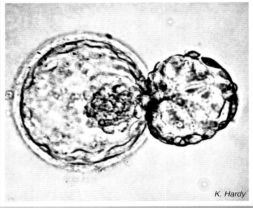

K. Hardy

4. Blastocyst hatching out of zona

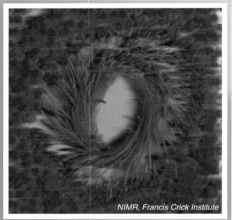

NIMR, Francis Crick Institute

5. Cross-section of seminiferous tubule where sperm are made; sperm heads in blue, tails in red

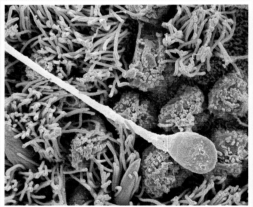

6. Single sperm cell

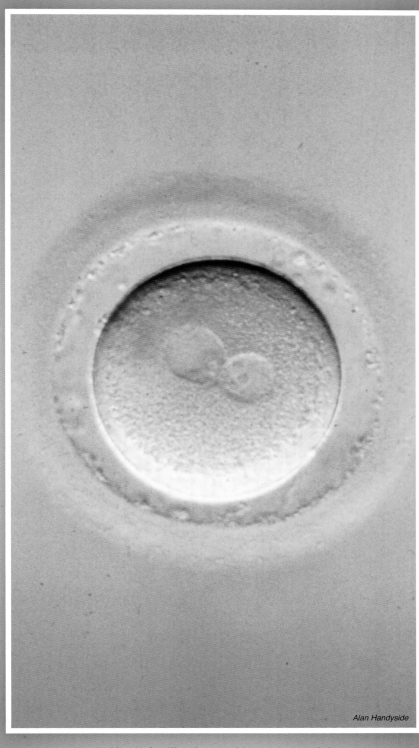

7. Newly fertilised egg with two pronuclei
clearly visible

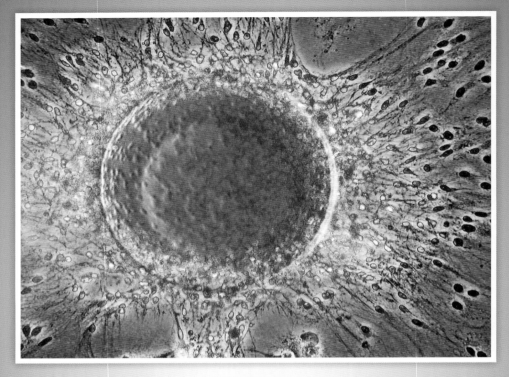

8. Fertilisation

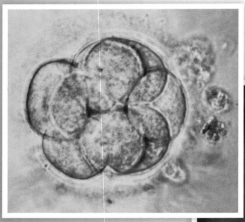

9. Embryo from IVF, 8 cells

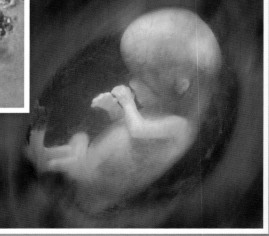

10. Embryo 10 weeks

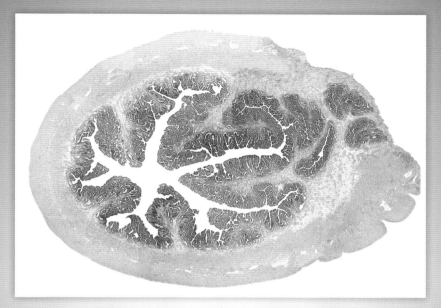

11. Cross section of oviduct or uterine tube

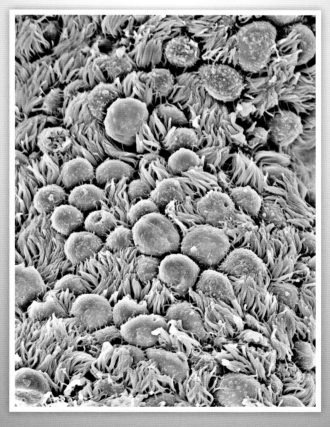

12. Lining of the uterine tube with villi clearly visible

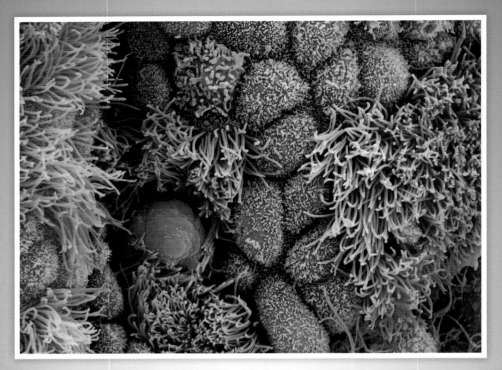

13. Ecosystem inside the uterine tube

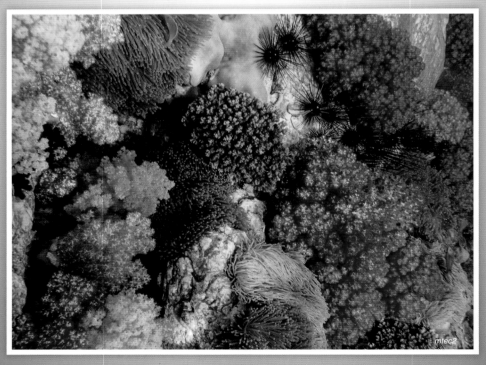

14. Coral reef

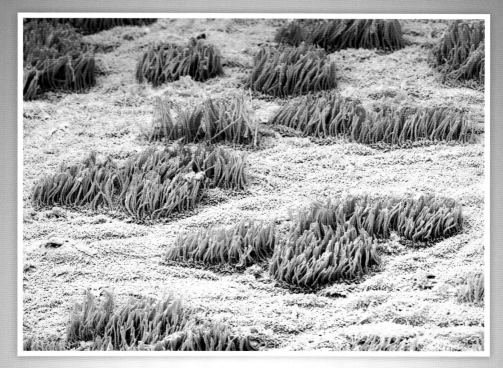

15. Endometrium – lining of the uterus

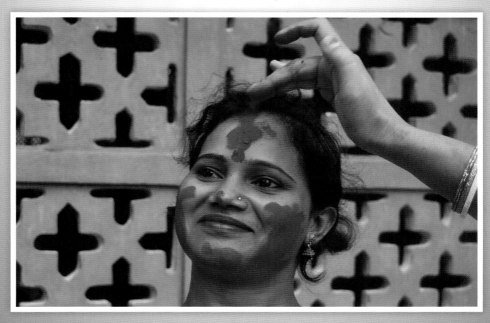

**16. Woman at Kharchi Puja festival in Tripura, India.
Ritual face painting with vermilion, celebrating the menstruation
of Mother Earth.**

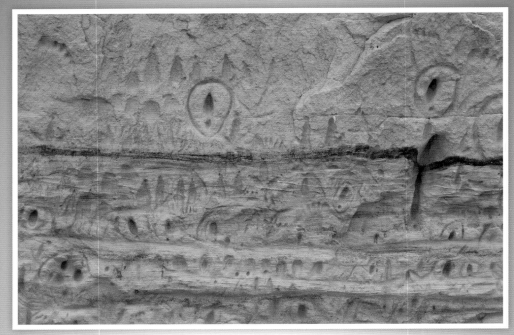

**17. Carved Aboriginal cave art of vulva,
Carnarvon Gorge, Qld, Australia**

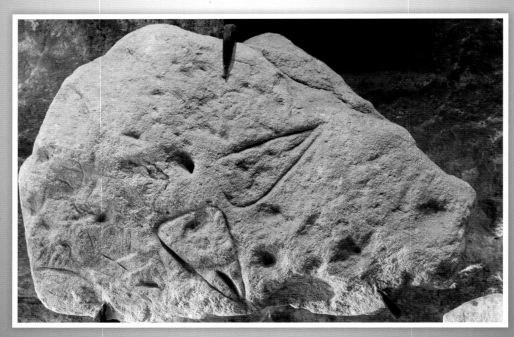

18. Cave art of engraved vulva, France, 30,000BC

Although only about 2cm long, the cervix is an incredibly sensitive part of our erotic anatomy with a whole plexus of nerves in the surrounding tissues that provide very pleasurable sensations during deep vaginal penetration. There's also a powerful energetic connection between the heart and the cervix, between love and pleasure, between heart-action (courage) and birthing.

The design of the cervix is really interesting because it's not simply an extension of the uterine muscles; it's actually made from different tissue, mainly dense connective tissue that's interspersed with muscle fibres (similar to the structure of the penis). Connective tissue has unique properties that distinguish it from muscle. In particular, it's comprised of what's called an **extracellular matrix**, which surrounds the living cells of the tissue. This matrix structure enables the cervix to bear weight, to withstand pressure and to endure physical stress that muscle could not. This is how it bears the weight of a baby during pregnancy and the physical extremes of dilation and expulsion during labour.

Paradoxically, at the same time, through a delicate series of gland-like folds, the cervix also produces the vital mucus secretions that are essential for fertilisation and conception. With a perfect female blend of strength and softness, the cervix is thus both 'iron woman' and 'juice maker'!

Cervical Mucus

Instead of just one secretion, cervical mucus is a sophisticated series of secretions that's so ingenious it deserves some detailed examination. Let's see how it works. Lining the endocervical canal are 100 or so gland-like crypts (Figure 6.4). These are actually oblique folds

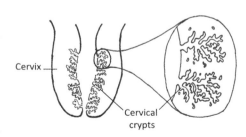

Figure 6.4

in the lining of the cervix, rather than true mucus-producing glands. These cervical crypts slope downwards and are continually secreting mucus into the vagina. [3]

Cervical mucus is vital to female fertility. We produce a healthy 20–60ml a day (1–2 tablespoons), often much more around ovulation. Many women have told me they sought medical advice because they thought their profuse 'discharge' was a symptom of infection. On the contrary, this is a healthy sign of fertility! However, when a discharge smells offensive, is itchy or has a peculiar colour (greenish or yellow), it's an indication of infection or disease, and it's important to seek medical attention.

As we've already seen, cervical mucus provides the transport for sperm to travel through the cervix and up into the tubes. In the 1950s, Professor Eric Odeblad[4] and his colleagues at the University of Umea in Sweden identified three different types of cervical mucus, produced in three different types of crypts: (Figure 6.5)

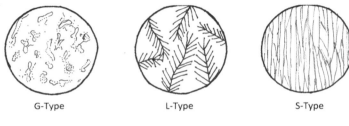

G-Type   L-Type   S-Type

Figure 6.5

1. **G-type** – Early in the cycle after menstruation when oestrogen levels are low, the mucus is scant, tacky and opaque; G-type mucus is comprised largely of protein fibres and forms a barrier to sperm.

2. **L-type** – As oestrogen levels rise towards ovulation, the mucus increases in amount, becoming thinner and milkier, sometimes with a lumpy texture; L-type mucus replaces G-type and has a number of important functions:

   • it's alkaline, which is vital if sperm are to survive in the acidic ph of the vagina

   • it traps defective sperm by directing them into an L-secreting unit and holding them there

   • it provides structural support for the third type of mucus: S-type

3. **S-type** – When oestrogen levels peak just before ovulation, the mucus becomes clear and runny, with the characteristic consistency of raw egg-white. This glossy, super-fertile mucus is beautifully named **spinnbarkeit** (a German word related to spider's web) because of its capacity to stretch into a delicate strand centimetres long.

The impenetrable G-mucus is formed in the lowest one-fifth of the cervical canal near the external opening; L-mucus is produced in the largest area of the endo-cervix, in crypts alternating with S-mucus; and S-mucus is produced in the highest crypts, deep in the endo-cervical canal.

Around ovulation, mucus quantity is up to *ten times* greater than earlier in the cycle! This fertile mucus creates a beautiful, slippery, lubricative sensation around the vulva which can be quite arousing. It displays a lovely 'ferning' pattern when viewed under a microscope, thought to be caused by channels in the S-type mucus

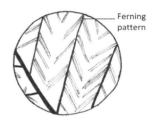

Ferning pattern

Figure 6.6

itself. (Figure 6.6) These channels create an ingenious kind of biological valve that supports sperm to make their way up through the cervix to the uterine tubes to find the egg. Supported by a scaffolding of L-type mucus, the S-mucus channels number up to 400 around ovulation! As you can see, this is a complex and sophisticated design.

Odeblad's research showed that the absence of these S-mucus channels prevents sperm from making their way into the uterus and is one of the major causes of female infertility. Odeblad also found that the cervical crypts producing these different types of mucus change significantly across the lifespan and under the influence of hormonal contraception. Young women typically have a proliferation of S-crypts, while premenopausal women have fewer. By design, the S-crypts undergo a normal process of transformation into L-crypts, which is amazingly reversed during pregnancy. For women on the Pill, however, the change to L-crypts is accelerated, with significant repercussions for their fertility. According to Odeblad:

"... a pregnancy rejuvenates the cervix by 2–3 years, but for each year the Pill is taken, the cervix ages by an extra year. If a woman takes the Pill for 10–15 years and then ceases taking it in order to achieve pregnancy, she may encounter some difficulties. Studies indicate that the number of S crypts are very few and, as well, the cervical canal will be very narrow." [5]

Prolonged use of the Pill can cause the sensitive S-crypts to atrophy. In my practice, I've witnessed fertility problems in women wanting to conceive in their late 30s after having been on the Pill for a decade or more. A number of measures can support the cervix to regain its function. Evening primrose oil has been shown to foster cervical mucus production, as has the amino acid L-Arginine. Some herbal treatments can also be effective, so it's worth consulting a good herbalist. In addition, a product called *Pre-Seed*, a 'fertility-friendly' personal lubricant developed by a female physiologist, mimics S-type mucus and facilitates sperm transport.

Sperm can linger in cervical mucus crypts nourished by factors in the fertile mucus and emerge hours or even days later. This explains how conception can occur up to five days after a single act of lovemaking. Following ovulation, the mucus very quickly reverts to the non-fertile G-type under the influence of progesterone. It becomes thick, tacky and impenetrable to sperm, forming a barrier at the external cervical opening.

This detailed knowledge about mucus changes around ovulation is crucial for couples wanting to conceive. When you see and sense the presence of L-type and especially the abundant, luscious S-type mucus, that's the perfect time for lovemaking. S-type mucus is at its most fertile about 24hrs *before* ovulation. This is Nature's way of ensuring that sperm will have time to swim up to the outer third of the tube, so they are capacitated, ready and waiting for the egg to be released.

As you can see, the cervix like the entire uterus, displays mobility, diversity, complexity and flexibility that are truly awe-inspiring. These qualities are magnified in the following section, which looks in detail at the function of the uterus.

FUNCTIONS OF THE UTERUS

The uterus is designed to receive, hold and nourish a fertilised egg, grow the embryo into a baby and then push the baby out at full-term. Given these functions, both the initial and final stages of the process – implantation and birth – are critical periods. The astonishing manner in which the uterus accomplishes these tasks, its interaction with the nesting embryo and its final act of birthing the baby, reveal the exceptional power and strength of the womb. Let's now explore them in detail.

Implantation

As we saw in Chapter Two, implantation occurs about seven days after fertilisation, when the fertilised egg has made its way down the tube and grown to a sufficient stage of maturity to burrow in. We tend to think of this as an easy and inevitable process, yet in fact, there's only a small window of opportunity when this is possible because the uterus is receptive to implantation for just a brief interval each cycle.

For a period of about 36 hours, which coincides *exactly* with the time when the morula would reach the uterus, a reciprocal relationship exists between this tiny organism and the mother's endometrium. The process of implantation is an intimate dialogue between the two. Here's what happens. The morula firstly imbibes some uterine fluid and it's this liquid that forms the fluid-filled central cavity of the blastocyst. As the zona pellucida thins and hatches, the cells of the blastocyst are exposed. The outer wall of the developing embryo, the **trophoblast** (*'nourishment generator'*), now discerningly tests the readiness of the endometrium for its receptivity to implantation. When it finds a site with the right chemical signals, the blastocyst anchors itself by secreting digestive enzymes that dissolve a pathway into the endometrial tissue. The trophoblast now forms two distinct layers: (Figure 6.7)

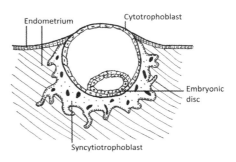

Figure 6.7

1. the **cytotrophoblast** (cyt = *cell*, tropho = *nourish*), the inner layer which retains its cell boundaries;

2. the **syncytiotrophoblast** (syn= *together*, cyt = *cell*), which sheds its cell membranes and penetrates right into the endometrium.

In this way, the blastocyst literally burrows into the uterine lining and is then surrounded by a pool of blood and glucose-laden cells, which provide a rich source of nourishment. This blood, which is shed during menstruation, is thus literally the cradle of life. Every human being who's ever existed began life in this cradle. Understanding the intimate dialogue between the blastocyst and the mother's endometrium enables us to appreciate the precious substance that becomes our menstrual blood each month.

What follows next is truly amazing! The surface layer of endometrial cells completely grows over the implantation site through a process known technically as 're-epithelialisation of the endometrial surface'. This means that during implant-ation, there's a complete sealing off of the blastocyst from the womb cavity. Just think about that for a moment! *The new organism is now totally absorbed into the womb lining, deep inside the mother's tissues!* (Figure 6.8)

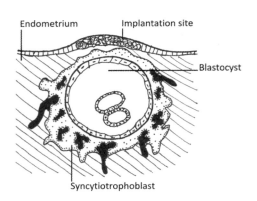

Figure 6.8

This profound boundary penetration could be considered the most intimate physical union possible between two human beings; the two have become literally one flesh. The absorption of the embryo into the womb lining defies the normal immune rejection governing all other body tissues. Hormonal signals from the embryo override this rejection response. And although the embryo and mother are fused together, each continues to exercise autonomous and independent contributions to the relationship. A dialogue is happening!

For its part, the trophoblast now begins to secrete the hormone **human chorionic gonadotropin (HCG)**, which instructs the corpus luteum in the ovary to continue secreting oestrogen and progesterone, thereby forestalling menstruation and maintaining the pregnancy. HCG is the pregnancy hormone detected in urine and blood tests in early pregnancy, a self-proclaiming message from the newly created organism that it exists and is present in the womb. The **chorion** (Greek khórion, *'membrane surrounding the fetus'*) which develops from the trophoblast, continues HCG production and in this way, the developing embryo takes over temporary hormonal control of the womb.

In response, the womb continues to nourish the growing embryo with its rich blood supply and store of glycogen (a carbohydrate stored in the endometrial cells), as well as forming a protective barrier right around it. By the second month, the placenta has taken over the functions of nourishment, oxygen supply and disposal of waste for the embryo; it also assumes the production of progesterone and oestrogen for the rest of the pregnancy.

Pregnancy

During pregnancy, there are some impressive changes in the structure of the uterus. The muscle layers increase in bulk by about 25 times! Eileen and Isidore Gersh describe this phenomenon in their book *The Biology of Women*:

> *"These increases are not simply an effect of stretching, as if it were a balloon, because the internal pressure remains virtually the same. The tremendous enlargement is achieved perhaps partly by an increase in number in the uterine muscle cells (perhaps due to increased progesterone in the maternal plasma) but mostly because of the increase in size of the uterine muscle cells due to higher levels of oestrogen in the maternal circulation. This is accompanied by increased formation of connective tissue and vascularity."* [6]

So we can see that even at a cellular level, the uterus displays incredible adaptability in carrying out its functions. It increases its mass and blood vessel supply by a huge amount to accommodate the demands of pregnancy. Its cleverness in adapting is further evident when we review the culminating moment of pregnancy, the outcome towards which all the preceding events have been geared: the birth of the new baby.

Birth or Parturition ('*bringing forth young*')

During labour and birth we see the uterus at its most powerful, tumultuous and mysterious. While the physiology is spectacular enough, the symbolic and spiritual significance of these events endow the uterus with a profoundly transformative potential. Here we see the boundary-penetration that characterises so much female embodiment at its absolute pinnacle.

Birth is sacred. Like death, it is the portal of life. During these threshold experiences, the veil between visible and invisible worlds thins, making Spirit more accessible. And it's the boundary penetration itself that makes this possible. During birth, it's not just a woman's womb and vagina that open to their absolute maximum; her whole being opens up during this time-stopping event. It's a period of exceptional vulnerability on all levels: body, mind, heart and spirit. For the sacredness of the moment to be safeguarded, respected and honoured, it's essential to choose caregivers and birth place wisely.

Whilst the precise mechanism that initiates labour is not yet known, the hormonal dialogue between mother and baby plays a vital role. The symbiotic relationship which began during implantation again becomes obvious with the onset of labour. This is how it happens. During the final weeks of pregnancy, oestrogen from the placenta peaks at its highest levels in the mother's bloodstream. This has two major effects:

1. It stimulates the myometrial cells to develop abundant **oxytocin** receptors; oxytocin is the hormone that stimulates contractions during labour.

2. It reduces progesterone's sedative effect on the myometrium, which then becomes increasingly active and begins to undergo irregular preparatory contractions, known as **Braxton Hicks contractions**, which are warm-ups for labour.

It is believed that the baby determines the end of the pregnancy. Given its self-directed intelligence as an organism from the very beginning, it's important to respect the baby's intelligence in signalling its readiness for birth. The baby prepares for birth by releasing cortisol, which helps its lung to mature, and a hormonal precursor for oestrogen produced in the placenta.[7] The mother too prepares for labour through rising oestrogen, cortisol and oxytocin levels, which stimulate the production and release of local hormones known as **prostaglandins**, which in turn stimulate the uterus. Thus a complex hormonal dance between mother and baby culminates in the onset of labour.

With the myometrium already sensitised to oxytocin, the combination of regular pulses of oxytocin from the pituitary, plus the action of prostaglandins and other factors, ensures that contractions become increasingly powerful. By now, the escalating sensations engage the mother's brain: her pituitary releases more oxytocin, as well as beta-endorphins for pain relief. A positive feedback loop begins – stronger contractions trigger the release of more oxytocin, which generates stronger contractions, which in turn stimulates more oxytocin. The great journey of labour is underway!

Stages of Labour

Although labour is conventionally divided into three stages, it's really one continuum that began at conception and continues on into breastfeeding and parenting. However it's useful to explore the process in phases, especially to appreciate the power of the uterus at different times in labour.

During the first stage, the energy movement in the uterus is to thicken the fundus and open the cervix. In the second stage, the energy movement changes to bearing the baby down the birth canal, while the third stage involves the birth of the placenta and membranes. The physiology, behaviour and shape of the uterus is different in each of these stages. It contracts differently, exerts force in different ways and alters its muscle proportions dramatically. So let's now explore each phase.

1. First Stage – Dilation of the cervix

This first stage of labour lasts from the beginning of surges (or contractions) until full dilation of the cervix. In my birth preparation sessions, I encourage the mother to relax as much as possible during this phase, so all her energy can go to her womb, which is undergoing an extraordinary transformation of its shape and structure. This is a time of turning deep within, of increased introspection and letting go her social brain and the externals, so her attention is focussed on releasing, relaxing and surrendering to the transformation process inside her body.

Physiologically, what happens in this stage is that the long muscle fibres of the myometrium progressively shorten in a process of **retraction**. Normally when muscles contract in other parts of the body, they subsequently return to their former length. By contrast, the myometrium fibres continue shortening without returning to their previous length. (Figure 6.9) As a result, the uterine wall thickens from 6mm at the start to about 25mm at the end, a significant change. Each contraction begins in the region of the tubes and fundus, then spreads down over the uterus. The effect of the upper region shortening and thickening is that the lower part thins and opens.

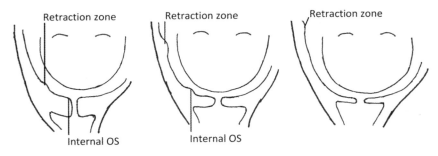

Figure 6.9

During this stage, the main action of the myometrium is creating thickness at the fundus, so it can exert a piston-like action to push the baby down the birth canal during second stage labour. Simultaneously, the cervix draws open to its greatest stretch: an astonishing 10cm! This is full dilation. The stage is now set for the most active part of labour during which the mother plays a dynamic role in bearing her baby down.

2. Second Stage –Bearing the baby down

The shift from first to second stage labour (sometimes called **transition**) is marked by significant changes in the energy movement and action of the uterus. Instead of an upward-pulling shortening of the vertical muscles, the action now shifts to a strong, downward expulsion. This dramatic turnaround can be disorienting for a labouring woman because it can seem as if everything has suddenly changed, so it's helpful to understand what's happening.

The reason for this shift is physiological. As the baby's head passes out of the cervix, it leaves a space in the uterus, so the vertical muscles need to retract to become snug around the baby again. There's often a lull while this takes place. Then, as the baby's head descends into the top of the vagina, it creates a big distension of the vaginal tissues, prompting a surge of oxytocin which initiates the bearing-down reflex.

During this transition, the mother may need time to adjust to the new sensations without pressure. If she's supported patiently, she'll move into her active participation in birthing her baby. As she works with the expulsive surges to bear her baby down her vagina, she'll instinctively choose positions that are conducive, so she can most effectively work with the contractions. Upright postures enable gravity to support the baby's descent and if she tunes into her body and her baby, she'll know what feels best for her.

These bearing-down surges engage the mother's whole body, not just her uterus. Her abdominal muscles and internal organs, her arms and legs, her neck and facial muscles, everything, is caught up in the often overwhelming urge to bear down. During this stage, women have a large increase in adrenaline and noradrenaline fuelling their energy and they sometimes report feeling very powerful. After hours of surrendering to the cervical *s-t-r-e-t-c-h*, they can now play an active role in bringing forth their babies. The hard work implicit in the term 'labour' now comes into its own. In second stage labour, women's bodies do the hardest physical work of which they're capable. Bearing down can be purely involuntary, rather than deliberate pushing.

With each expulsive downward surge, the baby's head moves towards the vaginal opening, drawing back slightly between surges. Finally the head presses fully into the vaginal opening and remains there, a moment called **crowning**. Like the astonishing stretch of the cervix, the vaginal opening, at the other end of the birth canal, is also superbly designed to stretch to allow first the baby's head and then the rest of the little body to come tumbling out.

In an undisturbed birth, peak hormone levels (oxytocin, beta-endorphins, prolactin and catecholamines) in both the mother's and the baby's bloodstreams prime them to experience the occasion as blissful, euphoric, even ecstatic.[8] Midwives and birthing mothers and fathers sometimes describe the special atmosphere that pervades the room just after a baby has been born. It's as if something eternal opens up in the space, touching them to their core. The magical moment when a child is born is said to change the very fabric of existence and the whole universe has to shift to make space for this new person.

3. Third Stage – Birth of the placenta

Once the infant is born, the process is brought to completion by the birth of the placenta and membranes. During this stage, the energy movement changes yet again. The womb contracts to compress its blood vessels and minimise blood loss, and also to detach the placenta from its inner surface. Once placenta and membranes are birthed, the uterus continues retracting and shrinking, an action facilitated by the first mother–baby interactions that lead to the onset of breastfeeding.

Breastfeeding involves the production of two hormones: **prolactin**, which stimulates milk production, and **oxytocin**, which is responsible for the 'let-down' (milk ejection) reflex. As we've seen, oxytocin stimulates uterine contractions, so when mothers put their babies to the breast immediately after birth, this is Nature's way of enabling the uterus to contract to prevent blood loss. These contractions can be quite strong, are sometimes uncomfortable, and usually subside after the first few hours of breastfeeding.

During subsequent days and weeks, the process by which the uterus returns to its pre-pregnant size is called **involution**. After having undergone the extremes of pregnancy, labour and birth, the womb now sets about restoring itself with characteristic ingenuity. Involution is caused by a phenomenon at the cellular level known as **autolysis**, a mechanism of self-digestion by the cell, where enzymes break down excess cytoplasm, and blood vessels that are no longer needed degenerate.

Amazingly, by about the tenth day after birth, the endometrium has regenerated, except for the placental site, which takes another six weeks to heal over completely. The blood flow after childbirth, known as the **lochia**, consists of blood, cells, tissues and blood vessels; it has quite a sweet smell which differs from that of menstrual blood. Lochia lasts for 2–4wks and can stop and start again for some time after this. After giving birth, the uterus doesn't quite return to its pre-pregnant dimensions and remains slightly larger than before.

The uterus is truly a force of nature, a mysterious space that is beyond our capacity to comprehend and that deserves our total respect. Given its extravagant expansion during pregnancy, the stretching and significant changes in shape and proportion during labour, and the incredible expulsive power involved in birthing a baby, it seems extraordinary that this amazing organ can return to its small inverted pear shape and resume its quiescent position inside the pelvis – until the next pregnancy. And that it can perform this creative feat over and over and over again. I am full of admiration for the wombs of our predecessors who gave birth to big families of ten children or more.

Symbolism of the Uterus

In ancient times and in many tribal cultures today, the womb is seen as the seat of power and authority for a woman. Anyone who has ever witnessed or experienced a birth will appreciate the awesome power of the uterus. It is the exultant power of pure femaleness. As cradle of life, the womb is truly an alchemical space in which a miraculous transformation occurs; a tiny fertilised egg, over the course of 40 weeks, develops into a totally new human being, who is then birthed into the world.

This alchemical space still exists inside women who've had a hysterectomy because of the holographic template (described in Chapter Three) upon which the third-dimensional organ rests. The alchemy of the uterus may involve a physical baby or something else. In *Women's Anatomy of Arousal*, Sheri Winston describes the womb's capacity to alchemically create 'the gold of new life':

"Whether it's a tiny new being, a work of art or a revolutionary vision, yin magic is at work when we receive inspiration, cook it inside and birth our new creation into the world." [9]

Curiously, the male counterpart to this female power is the erect phallus, a parallel brought home to me by a sculpture at an exhibition by Brisbane artist and doctor, Susan Byth. The sculpture featured a uterus and phallus, mounted horizontally centimetres apart, with the cervix facing the head of the phallus. Seeing these organs poised in salute to one another provoked an instant recognition: the archetypal female power of the uterus finds its match in the archetypal male power of the phallus. When I asked Susan about the inspiration for the piece, she said she'd been doing a Pap smear one day at her medical practice and the woman's cervix, drizzling glossy cervical mucus, reminded her of a phallus oozing semen.

This is the point at which male and female are profoundly different. Despite the embryonic similarities of the common genital tubercle, and the dual reproductive duct systems, female and male are not simply analogues of one another. Males don't possess anything remotely resembling a uterus; females, even though they possess erectile genital structures which derive from the same tissues as male genitals, do not demonstrate the male prowess of the erect phallus. Uterus and phallus embody two discrete potencies, each one unique to their sex and very different from the other.

Womb energy confers qualities of receptivity, creativity, forbearance, transformation, courage, commitment and cosmological power. The uterus actively receives, drawing in the raw ingredients of life. It is gestational and incubating. It holds and preserves, protects and nourishes. The womb possesses enormous elasticity and adaptability. It absorbs new life and negotiates major readjustments so that that new life can come into being. Then, when the time has come, the uterus transforms from soft, receptive, accommodating and expanding into hard, contracting, expulsive and ejecting. It expels new life with tremendous force and implacability. Here again we see the paradox of female strength.

Womb as Sacred Symbol

The uterus fills and empties each month with menstruation. It also fills and continues to fill during pregnancy. As it fills, the womb 'gives matter to'. The word 'mother' derives from the Latin *materia*, meaning 'substance' or 'matter'. The womb is the place where what once existed in spirit now finds substance and form. Jamie Sams, a French Native American midwife and teacher, describes this process well:

> *"Women give birth to their dreams through their womb... Let's say you have this wonderful idea, and there it is in the thought universe ... How do you make that idea manifest in physical reality? You bring it down from the sky into the earth... if you want to bring the dream into being, you use this beautiful body that you have been given to walk it, to take action, to make it happen."* [10]

As symbol of the sacred, the womb perfectly expresses the embodied nature of female spirituality. As females, we 'give matter' not only to our physical babies, but to all manner of creative outpourings, whether they be artistic endeavours, innovative policies, career projects or the quality of our lives. In handling blood, secretions, milk, regurgitated food, soiled nappies and the messiness of creation, we take in the raw ingredients of life and weave miracles. I believe that within the sacred space of our womb lies the Divine Matrix,[11] our energetic connection to the source of Life itself. Interestingly, the word 'matrix' derives from the Latin for 'womb'.

The uterus is one of the most active, creative, dynamic and powerful organs in a woman's body. It's a place of extremes and contradictions. It opens and closes, contracts, dilates, hardens, softens, stretches, retracts, thickens, thins, balloons, shrinks, draws in and pushes out. It displays both wondrous powers of incubation and truly awesome powers of expulsion. The uterus is without doubt the female symbol *par excellence.*

Reflection

What I now know about my uterus that I didn't know before is…

What I most love and appreciate about my uterus is…

When I reflect on this information, what strikes or moves me is…

Affirmation

I love the creative power of my womb. It is the Cradle of Life and I honour its Sacred Covenant.

Suggestion

Lie down on your belly on the ground for 15mins. Feel the magnetic support of Earth beneath you. Ask Earth to align your womb with the energetic force field of Her molten magma core. Pour out your heart, speak your concerns and then wait for Her response; it might come immediately or in the following hours or days. Do this practice regularly.

Chapter Seven

The Vagina

The **vagina** (*'sheath'*) is the beautiful passageway that connects our inner reproductive world with our outer world. Under-appreciated and often over-looked, the vagina is as intelligent, flexible and versatile as our other internal organs. It holds some delicious goodies in the pleasure department and is way more active than its name suggests.

Positioned between the urethra and bladder at the front and the rectum and anus at the back, the vagina is an elastic, fibro-muscular canal leading from the vulva to the cervix. (Figure 7.1) While the dimensions of the vagina in its resting state vary considerably from woman to woman, the 'average' textbook measurement is about 7.5cm for the vagina's front wall, with the back wall longer at about 10cm. (Figure 7.2) While most diagrams illustrate the vagina as an open tube, it's really a *potential* cavity with its front and back walls touching each other.

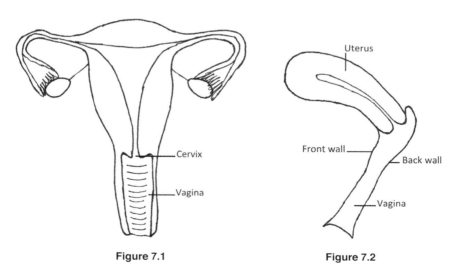

Figure 7.1

Figure 7.2

The vagina has a number of anatomical subdivisions. The **vaginal orifice** is the external opening into the vulva and just inside this is the **vaginal corona**, comprised of stretchy tissue forming a crown-shape. Previously known as the **hymen** ('*membrane*'), the corona was renamed in 2009 by a Swedish sexual rights group to dispel the myth of the hymen as the 'boundary between guilt and innocence'.[1] Rather than a membrane that can be ruptured, it's actually a ring of membranous folds of tissue in a variety of configurations. (Figure 7.3) As a remnant of fetal development, the corona remains part of our anatomy for life. Beyond the corona is the **vaginal canal** which widens at the end to encompass the cervix, an area known as the **vaginal vault**.

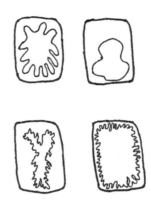

Figure 7.3

To appreciate the true beauty of the vagina, we need to look more closely at its design which has some unexpectedly marvellous features. The structure of the vaginal walls is comprised of three layers: (Figure 7.4)

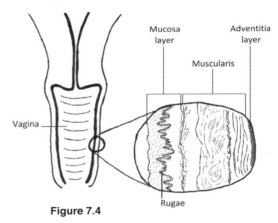

Figure 7.4

1. an internal **mucosa** layer (mucus lining) which features some horizontal folds called **rugae** ('*ridges*')

2. a middle **muscularis** layer of smooth muscle fibres, with an inner circular layer and an outer longitudinal one (similar to the uterus and tubes)

3. an external **adventitia** layer of dense, fibro-elastic connective tissue that's rich in collagen and has great powers of distension

The middle muscle layer is supplied with nerves from the autonomic nervous system, which means that it's controlled by the subconscious. Amazingly, this smooth muscle layer contains at least 14 different neurotransmitters (chemicals that communicate across nerve synapses), including dopamine, noradrenaline, oxytocin and relaxin.[2] While the exact function of each neurotransmitter during sexual arousal is unknown, it seems that some of them support vaginal lubrication and it's likely that others are related to our pleasure potential.

The vagina's inner mucus lining also does some clever things. It consists of two layers:

1. the **inner epithelium**, a constantly-shedding protective layer approximately 30 cells deep, designed to accommodate penetration

2. the **lamina propria** (*'thin plate'*), a layer of connective tissue containing elastic fibres that return the vagina to its original shape after expansion

The vaginal epithelium is extremely responsive to oestrogen, so as oestrogen levels rise during the menstrual cycle, the epithelium grows into multiple layers. As the epithelial cells grow, they continually shed into the vaginal cavity, along with a moist layer of **glycocalyx** (*'sugar cup'* – what a gorgeous name!), a carbohydrate-rich substance found at the cell surface. These discarded cells are then acted upon by friendly micro-organisms (called **Doderlein's bacilli**), which convert the glycogen to lactic acid. This mechanism ensures that the ph of the vagina remains acidic (3.5 to 4ph), a necessity given its roles.

Through this brilliant design, the vagina is continually self-cleansing, adjusting its internal medium to allow boundary penetration without the risk of constant infection. Whilst the womb is not designed to withstand an influx of micro-organisms, the vagina is well adapted to do so. As its purpose is to mediate between outside and inside, it contains friendly organisms and lactic acid to ensure bacteria coming from outside don't proliferate. The ingenuity of this design can be compromised by things like 'feminine hygiene' products, which interfere with the efficiency of these processes.

Functions of the Vagina

Despite its unassuming profile, the vagina has many significant functions:

1. it's an outlet for uterine secretions – cervical mucus and menstrual flow

2. it's the female organ for penetrative sex, with amazing pleasure potential

3. it provides optimum access to the cervix for sperm

4. it's the birth canal

Each of these functions yields some wonderful secrets, so let's explore further.

1. Outlet for uterine secretions

We've already seen how the alkalinity of fertile cervical mucus in the vagina is vital to sperm survival and transport through the cervical canal into the uterus. Well there's also a clever feature regarding cervical mucus at the lower end of the vagina too. At its base, the vagina is supported by the pelvic floor muscles, which wrap like a figure-eight around the vagina, urethra and anus. Just above this muscle layer inside the vagina are the **paraurethral pockets** (the Pockets of Shaw), small recesses extending from the vagina on each side of the urethra. In another clever design feature, the cells in these pockets are specially modified to secrete manganese, which by a simple chemical reaction, reabsorbs water and electrolytes from the mucus.

This neat housekeeping gesture is again dependent upon oestrogen. With higher oestrogen levels just prior to ovulation, manganese secretion is inhibited by a 'waterproofing' of the vaginal epithelium. This allows the fertile, egg-white cervical mucus to make its way down to the vulva, thereby facilitating sperm survival. After ovulation, the paraurethral pockets resume their release of manganese and the water and electrolytes in the mucus are again reabsorbed. This intriguing capacity of the vagina is little guessed at, even by medical professionals.

Menstrual flow, the other uterine secretion, will be examined in detail in Chapter Nine about menstruation.

2. The Female Organ for Penetrative Sex

As a sexual organ, the vagina is often described passively as simply a receptacle for a penis. Our magnificent female apparatus, its agency and what's available to us through this organ deserve better naming. The unfortunate origins of the word are described by Sheila Kitzinger:

> *"The term 'vagina' comes from the Latin for 'sheath' or 'scabbard'. This male encoding represents the vagina as a passive receptacle awaiting penetration as a scabbard awaits a sword. If women had the power to name and give meanings, the images associated with the vagina might well be much more active, creative and strong."* [3]

The male encoding of female anatomy has meant that many of our body parts were named after the male scientists who first described them. For example, the Fallopian tubes, Bartholin's glands, the Gräfenberg spot, the Mullerian ducts, the Pockets of Shaw, Braxton Hicks contractions, and so on. Because words are such powerful shapers of consciousness, I've avoided using these terms, preferring the Latin derivatives, which often contain interesting meanings.

Consider the symbolism of this male naming of the vagina for a moment. What's the function of a sheath or scabbard? It exists only to contain and protect the sword, no other purpose. The sword is the primary entity, the thing that acts. It can exist and function without the scabbard. Yet the scabbard's sole purpose is dependent upon the sword; its existence would be meaningless without it.

Note the analogy here. Many women struggle to find their sexual identity as something in its own right, *without reference to the sexual needs of men.* When an entire culture assigns meaning to something, as it does to women's sexual anatomy by the use of the term 'vagina', this has repercussions for our ability to perceive and experience our sexual identity, as it is in itself, with no external reference. Our culture has hoodwinked us about this, so the journey into an inner referenced sexual awareness and experience is essential for our autonomy.

As anyone who possesses a vagina can tell you, it's much more than a passive receptacle waiting for something outside to give it meaning! The vagina is an intimate part of our anatomy through which we experience and express who we are as a sexual being. Allowing admission to our inside-body-space, it exemplifies our capacity for boundary penetration as a source of pleasure, connection and the creation of new life. It deserves a much more proactive word to reflect its role as our sex organ. As we shall see, like the rest of our reproductive system, the vagina is wonderfully active, even at a cellular level, and although it's an organ of reception, this is a very *active* receptivity.

As the place of intromission, the vagina is beautifully crafted to maximise female sexual pleasure *under the right circumstances*. The spongy pad of tissue between the front of the vagina and the urethra, the **urethral sponge**, and the spongy pad between the vagina and the rectum, the **perineal sponge**, are made of erectile tissue which engorges during sexual arousal. (Figure 7.5) (The vestibular bulbs, which are also erectile tissue, will be described in the next chapter on the vulva.)

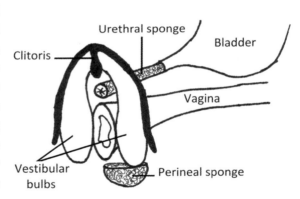

Figure 7.5

Sensations of engorgement by these erectile bodies – tingling, increased blood flow, turgidity and plumping of the tissues – provide the right circumstances to make penetrative sex pleasurable. More about this in the next chapter!

During sexual arousal, the vagina dramatically changes its shape, position and secretions. With a rich network of nerves and blood vessels that swell with stimulation, the vagina creates its own lubrication. Fluid from the swollen blood vessels oozes through the connective tissue and epithelium of the vaginal walls, providing that luscious wetness we recognise when aroused. (This wetness has a different origin to the wet sensation caused by fertile mucus from the cervix.)

Engorgement by the erectile tissues surrounding the vagina also causes an expansion in length and diameter inside the vagina. The dramatic changes brought about by increased blood flow during arousal are captured by Sheila Kitzinger:

> *"When we blush, feel self-conscious and go pink, our faces do not radically change their shape. The equivalent flow of blood to the vagina, however, results in a plumping up and opening which is more like a bud bursting into full flower."* [4]

Deep inside the vagina is a zone with potential for a completely different kind of pleasure than the clitoris. In the circular region around the outside of the cervix, there's a plexus of pelvic nerves, which are different to the nerve supply reaching the external genitals (the pudendal nerve). These pelvic nerves, which also branch into the uterus and anus, enter the vagina on each side of the vaginal vault behind the cervix and provide deep sensations of pleasure with their own unique quality. This zone is really responsive to deep thrusting, as long as a woman is highly aroused and the cervix has pulled up out of the way. When I access this space, I feel like I'm touching some of the deepest mysteries of the Universe, a cauldron of creative fire, intense heat and pleasure. This transcendent quality may also have something to do with the abundance of neurotransmitters mentioned earlier.

The Goddess Spot or G-spot

The G-spot is not really a spot but a highly sensitive region in the urethral sponge which can be felt along the front wall of the vagina. First documented in the 1950s by German physician, Ernst Von Grafenberg it was located at the place where the urethra joins the bladder. Grafenberg's identification and description of this sensitive area led researchers Beverly Whipple and John Perry to coin the term 'G-spot'. [5]

Just as the proportions of each woman's face are different, so too the specific location of the G-spot varies from woman to woman, depending upon her genital anatomy.[6] It may lie just inside the vaginal opening or be so deep that it's beyond finger reach, or anywhere in between. It typically has a slightly rougher, ribbed texture (more noticeable during arousal) than the rest of the urethral sponge. In contrast to the clitoris, it responds best to firm, rhythmic pressure on the roof of the vagina; a 'come hither' beckoning movement with the forefinger is perfect!

As described in their book, *The G Spot*, Beverly Whipple, John Perry and Alice Kahn Ladas write:

> *"The G spot is probably composed of a complex network of blood vessels, the paraurethral glands and ducts, nerve endings, and the tissue surrounding the bladder neck. In those women examined by us (or by others and reported to us), this sensitive area swelled with stimulation and the soft tissue began to feel hard, with well defined edges."*[7]

Embryologically, the G-spot is formed from the same tissue that becomes the prostate in men, so it's sometimes referred to as the female prostate. Because of its proximity to the urethra, stimulation of the G-spot can induce a sensation of needing to pee, even when the bladder is empty; this passes as sensations of pleasure increase. Stimulating our G-spot expands the sensual pleasure accessible to us in our vagina and opens the door to the possibility of female ejaculation.

Female Ejaculation

During prolonged stimulation of the urethral sponge, women may ejaculate a clear watery fluid with a faint musky odour. Some women are natural ejaculators, others learn to 'squirt', and all women have the necessary apparatus. Ejaculate may come out as a trickle, a gush or in strong expulsive splashes! And while it most commonly occurs during orgasm, it can also appear during deep arousal and is associated with wonderful feelings of pleasure and emotional satisfaction.

To date, there's insufficient scientific evidence to reliably determine the source of female ejaculate. Several small studies by male doctors have proposed that the fluid comes from the bladder (minus urea and creatinine which usually characterise urine) or that it may originate in the kidneys[8], or that it's urine.[9] Women ejaculators say it has a different smell and taste from urine. Sheri Winston maintains that the fluid comes from the **paraurethral glands** in the urethral sponge. Like the mucus ducts in the cervix, a network of tubules weaves through the urethral sponge, ending in about 30 ducts that open into the urethra.[10] (Figure 7.6) Research has shown two substances present in much higher levels in female ejaculatory fluid:

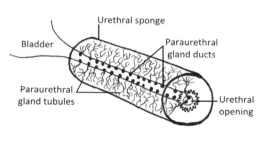

Figure 7.6

tartrate-inhibited acid phosphatase and glucose.[11] Studies have also found that ejaculate contains enzymes similar to that found in male seminal fluid, though in much lesser quantities.

In Taoist and Tantric traditions, female ejaculate is considered very sacred and was collected for ceremonies as a blessing. **Amrita** ('*nectar of life*') or **ambrosia,** as it's sometimes called, is also renowned for its medicinal properties and for inducing sensations of wellbeing and bliss in those who imbibe it. Expressing the exuberance of the vagina, these waters of life reflect a luscious, exultant celebration of the wetness that characterises so much female body experience.

As you can see, far from being merely a passive receptacle, the vagina possesses some very dynamic pleasure centres, with a much more active role than what's conveyed by the word 'sheath'. However, as a sheath, the vagina can also provide a protective boundary where unwanted energies coming in through penetration are contained, rather than diffusing throughout our bodies.

3. Optimum Access to the Cervix for Sperm

Prior to female orgasm, the part of the vagina nearest to the vulva swells markedly, reducing the diameter of the vagina, with a consequent 'hugging' on the penis during sex. This is known as the **orgasmic platform** and it alters the shape of the vagina so that its cervical end undergoes a kind of 'tenting' effect, enabling semen to pool in close proximity with the cervix. This tenting sometimes creates an anticipatory hollow or aching sensation, just prior to climax.

During orgasm, the orgasmic platform contracts rhythmically, as does the vulva, the womb, the rectum, the perineum and pelvic muscles. The cervix opening displays a sucking motion that helps to draw seminal fluid up inside the uterus. Without ongoing stimulation, the orgasmic platform returns to its non-aroused state, followed by a relaxation of the vaginal walls which shorten and decrease in diameter. With continuing stimulation, engorgement of the erectile tissues in the vagina can continue to provide hours of pleasure. Vaginal pleasure is also one of the best kept secrets of birthing in our culture, something we now explore in more detail.

4. The Birth Canal

The magnificence of the vagina really comes into its own during the birth process. With its exceptional powers of distension and elasticity, the vagina can easily accommodate the entire body of an infant during birth. Next time you see a newborn baby, notice how big that baby's dimensions are in comparison to the normal 1.5–2cm width of a vagina! The flexibility that allows the downward passage and birth of a baby, weighing over 3kg and roughly 25cm long, is truly astonishing.

Pregnant women often wonder how on earth something so big can emerge out of an opening so small. Especially for first time mothers, there's an almost universal fear of being split open, which can generate anxiety and apprehension. Some of these fears are a normal part of confronting the unknown; there's a part of our mind which cannot fathom how such a stretch is possible. Yet, our body and in particular our vagina, is superbly designed to negotiate exactly that kind of stretch.

During the expulsive second stage of labour, the baby's head causes the concertina-like folds of the vagina to fan out, gradually opening up the birth canal to accommodate the baby's body. When a woman is encouraged to find her own instinctive way of doing this, it can become an intensely sexual experience. In the hospital context, where there's no privacy and birth is generally associated with pain, this may come as a big surprise. Yet, the vagina's design is geared towards pleasure during birth.

As the baby's head descends towards the vaginal outlet, it puts pressure on the legs of the clitoris, the G-spot, and the urethral and the perineal sponges. Some women experience orgasmic sensations while this is happening and women have told me they felt embarrassed by their sexual sensations in such a public context. However, the design isn't faulty; it's our birthright to enjoy the pleasure our vagina provides at one of the most powerful times of our life. The sensations in the vagina and all the surrounding tissues, including the rectum and anus, and the powerful bearing down surges of second stage labour, all contribute to what can be an orgasmic experience.

This sensuality can also be a profoundly spiritual experience. As Sheila Kitzinger describes it:

"Suddenly she is full, stretched to her utmost, as if she is a seed-pod bursting. There is a moment of waiting, of awe, of a kind of tension which occurs just before orgasm and then suddenly the baby passes through, the whole body slips out in a rush of warm flesh, a fountain of water, a peak of overwhelming surprise and the little body is against her skin, kicking against her thighs or swimming up over her belly." [12]

The moment when a baby is poised to cross the threshold into the outside world can be full of mystery. Excited parents often describe the wonder of seeing a crescent of the baby's head at the vaginal opening, the face still veiled, yet their meeting imminent. The vagina shrouds it in mystery until the moment of birth when suddenly the new little person tumbles out and is veiled no longer.

The experience of a new soul emerging from within your own body is profoundly moving. The physical sensations of a wet baby slithering out, the enormous relief of a mission accomplished, the overwhelming emotion, the exhilaration of meeting your newborn face to face and the awesome boundary penetration of this moment, all combine to make birth an opening of the gates of grace. We realise we are in the presence of something infinitely greater than ourselves. Through the sacrament of birth, the space becomes sacred, the unseen hand of the divine touching all present.

During birth, the design of the vagina is flawless. The region around the vaginal opening is supplied with blood through very small vessels, so if a tear occurs during birthing, very little blood is lost. Two requirements are necessary to avoid tearing: 1) freedom from fear so the tissues can expand to their fullest without residual tension, and 2) no exhortation from others to 'push, push, push!' Vaginal tissues that are 'white-knuckling' with fear lose their elasticity, and pressure to push interferes with a woman's own timing.

After the birth, the muscular walls of the vagina retract and regain their former shape, usually with no permanent damage despite their enormous distension. This recovery is fostered by pelvic floor exercises, in which the vaginal and pelvic floor muscles are alternately squeezed, held and released to restore their tone and holding power. The common myth that vaginal birth will 'wreck' a woman's pelvic floor is based upon ignorance of the vagina's superb design and flexibility when unpressured.

Symbolism of the Vagina:

And the doorway of the Mysterious Female
Is the base from which Heaven and Earth sprang.
It is there within us all the while.

Tao Te Ching [13]

Symbolically the vagina is our gateway into the world. Despite rising caesarean rates, the vast majority of people make their entrance into life on Planet Earth through this the portal. The vagina is the mysterious doorway through which Spirit initiates its journey into matter, as well as the channel through which new life emerges nine months later. As Philip Sudo, author of *Zen Sex*, puts it:

> *"Remember, too, that just as we enter the world in a body, we enter the world through a body as well – the body of our mother. The vagina that's entered in sex is the same opening through which life enters the world; the point of entrance is the point of exit, and the point of all beginning."* [14]

In addition to being the 'point of all beginning', the vagina also has a lesser-known spiritual protective capacity. This protective power is graphically portrayed by the Sheela-na-Gig figure. (Figure 7.7) One translation of Sheela-na-Gig is 'vagina woman'. [15] The stone figures of Sheela with their wide open vaginas are found all over Ireland, Great Britain, France and Spain. Their prominent positioning up high on churches, castles

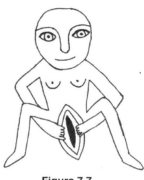

Figure 7.7

and other power spots is believed to repel evil spirits. Variations on the theme of the exposed vagina as a protective talisman warding off evil can be found in other parts of Europe, India, Indonesia and South America. As the sacred portal of life, it makes sense that the vagina would also protect that life from harm.

We can see from our exploration of the vagina that this remarkable endowment is vastly more substantial and active than a simple 'sheath'. At a cellular, muscular and functional level, the vagina displays the same ingenuity, flexibility, intelligence and versatility as so many of our other female organs. It bridges our inner and outer worlds with profound, life-changing consequences, as in the birth of a baby, and it expresses dimensions of our most intimate self in the sexuality of lovemaking.

Reflection

What I now know about my vagina that I didn't know before is...

What I most love and appreciate about my vagina is...

When I reflect on this information, what strikes or moves me is...

Affirmation

My vagina is the Gateway of Life. I love and appreciate its beauty.

Suggestion

Draw or paint a representation of the doorway of the Mysterious Female, the base from which Heaven and Earth sprang. When it's finished, place it on an altar with some flowers and sacred objects. Light a candle and pray a devotion of thanks for your sacred vagina.

Chapter Eight

❧

The Vulva

The external female genitals, known collectively as the **vulva** (*'covering'*), include a surprising array of different tissues, glands and structures: the mons pubis, the labia majora and labia minora, the clitoris, the vestibule of the vagina, the vaginal opening, the urethral outlet, the vestibular bulbs and the vestibular glands. As a sensing organ, the vulva has a vast and exquisite array of sensitive nerve endings and erectile structures, whose purpose is to bring us pleasure. In a moment we'll explore all the different aspects of this beautiful part of our anatomy.

Before we do, please note: *there is inexhaustible variety in the size, shape, colour and composition of female genitals.* So whatever your vulva looks like, it is perfectly normal and as unique as you are. As sex educator Emily Nagoski points out, we're all made from "the same parts, just organised in different ways". [1] The air-brushed versions shown in soft-porn magazines depict a version of the vulva without inner lips showing in order to meet legal requirements. Don't be fooled!

Many women feel ashamed of their genitals, believing them to be defective, unattractive or smelly. Nothing could be further from the truth. Our female genitals are one of the most beautiful and sacred places in our entire body. In parts of the world like India and Bali, carvings of female genitals adorn temple walls and holy sites, publicly venerating this part of the female body. I remember the joy I felt in first being exposed to these traditions.

In Western culture however, we grow up in a sex-negative atmosphere of shame and suppression about sexuality. Paradoxically, at the same time, the female body is sexualised as an object of gratification, used to sell things and demeaned with violence in pornography. This objectification and the cultural and religious shaming of female genitals, serves to disconnect us from our authentic sexuality and sexual power. And whose interests does that serve, I wonder? The good news is that because this shame is a social construction, we can deconstruct and transform it through knowledge and awareness. So hold that intent as you read this chapter.

To take ownership of the sacred power of our female genitals, we need to know its intimate terrain. Exploring the vulva is like entering a miniature universe full of wonders. As you study this chapter, have a mirror handy, preferably a magnifying one, so that you can see for yourself what your genital anatomy looks like. Let's now wander through the intricate features of our beautiful genitals, so we can truly appreciate them and enhance our capacity for pleasure.

Lying over the pubic bone is the soft, spongy rounded area covered with pubic hair known as the **mons pubis** (*'mountain on the pubis'*). Pubic hair is as variable as hair on the head in shape, amount and colour and although it's become popular to remove pubic hair, it does provide some cushioning on the pubic mound, as well as being sensitive to touch. It has another function too. The mons is well supplied with scent glands and pubic hair captures the aroma as a sexual cue for suitors!

The outermost covering of the vulva, the **labia majora** (*'larger lips'*), are the external folds of skin extending from the mons pubis at the front to the perineum at the back. (You might remember from Chapter Two that the labia majora derive embryologically from the same tissues that fuse together to become the male scrotum.) Their external surfaces are also covered with pubic hair, which is very sensitive to light touch. These outer lips enfold all the delicate inner structures of the vulva, which need protecting because of their exceptional sensitivity.

Within the outer lips are two soft, hair-free folds of skin called the **labia minora** (*'smaller lips'*), which extend from the hood of the clitoris to the perineum. Despite the literal translation of 'smaller lips', the labia minora in many women are larger than the outer lips and appear as succulent folds of flesh between the outer lips. (Embryologically they derive from the same tissue which forms the shaft of the male penis.) The inner lips are very smooth, highly sensitive tissues with a fine mucus membrane that's designed to stay moist or wet, like your eyeball; anything dry or rough will irritate. The labia minora are one of the most delightful, diverse and uniquely individual expressions of the beauty of our female genitals. Much like each flower has its own special arrangement of petals and colours, there's endless variety in the size, shape, colour and configuration of the inner lips, which are often asymmetrical. (Figure 8.1)

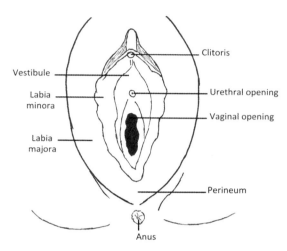

Figure 8.1

Within the labia minora is an area known as the **vestibule** (*'anteroom'*), which acts like a miniature ante-chamber to the vagina. Here we find several doorways, some juicy glands and some perfume outlets. At the top above the vagina (or sometimes just inside it) is the **urethral opening,** which is flanked by the **paraurethral gland ducts** (Skene's glands). (In the previous chapter, we looked at the paraurethral glands, the tubules in the urethral sponge that produce female ejaculate and open into the urethra; the paraurethral gland *ducts* are two slightly larger tubules that open into the vestibule at either side of the urethral outlet.)

Below the urethral outlet is the **vaginal opening**, either side of which are the **vestibular glands** (Bartholin's glands).These grape-sized glands opening into the vestibule are under-researched, so we don't yet know all their functions. What we do know is that they secrete mucus to keep the vulva moist and probably help maintain healthy genital ecology.[2] Along with vaginal lubrication and paraurethral gland secretions, they're also partly responsible for the wetness associated with sexual arousal.

The vestibule contains its very own perfume outlet, the **apocrine sweat glands**, responsible for the characteristic musky female genital aroma. Analogous to the scent glands of other mammals, their activity is increased by sexual excitement. They're known to enlarge and recede in harmony with the phases of the menstrual cycle, probably under the influence of oestrogen. Many women feel uncomfortable about the lovely smell of their genitals, so at the end of this chapter, I've suggested an activity to transform this discomfort.

At the top of the vestibule is the visible portion of the **clitoris** and at the bottom of the vestibule is the **perineum**, under which is the anus. The perineum is comprised of extremely elastic tissues and muscles, and the pelvic floor muscles are at their thickest here. During childbirth the perineum is designed to stretch enormously and if the baby's head is given time to crown gradually, the perineal tissues can remain completely intact.

THE CLITORIS: (*'little key'*)

As the meaning of the word suggests, the clitoris is a key to female pleasure. Many structures comprise the 'little key'. The **glans** (*'head'*) is the small visible portion at the tip of the **body** or **shaft**. In most women, both head and shaft are protected by a tent-like meeting of the labia minora, which forms a retractable hood over the glans. (In some women, the clitoris is not covered and the increased sensitivity often changes their arousal preferences.) If the hood is pulled back, the glans is clearly visible as a round pea-sized projection. The shaft which extends up from the glans towards the pubic bone, can be felt under the hood like a rubbery cord, roughly 2–5cm long. (Figure 8.2) At the end of

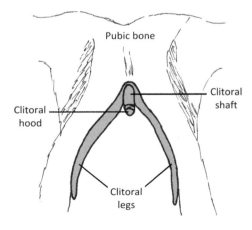

Figure 8.2

the shaft, the clitoris splits like a wishbone into two **crura** ('*legs*') about 9cm long, which flare out and back along the inner rim of the pubic arch. During arousal, the entire clitoris (glans, shaft and legs) becomes erect and hard.

Immediately below and between these two legs are the **vestibular bulbs**, two tear-shaped masses of erectile tissue that wrap either side of the vagina. The bulbs connect directly with the clitoral shaft at the top, so stimulation of either will impact both. Just as the clitoris changes shape when aroused, the vestibular bulbs plump up to almost double their size during arousal, making penetration feel wonderful.

The clitoris is really an exceptional organ, totally unique in its function. To appreciate this more fully, let's compare it to the penis. The penis has numerous functions: transporting urine from the bladder, the male organ for sexual intercourse, depositing sperm into the vagina, and the sensory organ of sexual pleasure for men. In contrast, the sole function of the clitoris is *sexual pleasure!* Nothing else! Just ponder this fact for a moment.

As females, Nature has endowed us with an organ whose only purpose is to bring us pleasure. This says something fundamental about female sexuality. Far from being merely adjuncts to male sexual needs, we possess our own pleasure architecture, expressly designed to *pleasure us*. The clitoral glans contains a staggering 8000 nerve endings! No other body part contains such a high concentration of nerve endings. It's so exquisitely sensitive that direct touch of the glans without lubrication is painful. From this remarkable design, we can be sure there's a very important contribution our pleasure can make in the world, or the Universe would never have invested such a high proportion of intelligent nerve endings in one place.

Erectile Structures of Female Arousal

The internal structure of the clitoral glans, shaft and legs is a maze of blood vessels and capillaries known collectively as the **corpus cavernosum** ('*body of caverns*'). The reason for this name becomes obvious during arousal when the inner chambers of these tissues fill with blood, which remains trapped there by valves. Simultaneously, a small ligament attached to the clitoral shaft from the pubic bone, draws the glans and shaft up, so the whole clitoris becomes erect, changing shape dramatically. (This tissue is homologous to the pair of cavernous bodies on either side of the penis and derives embryologically from the same tissue.)

In contrast, the urethral sponge, perineal sponge and vestibular bulbs are comprised of different tissue that engorges, rather than becomes erect, during arousal. This tissue, which is called the **corpus spongiosum** (*'spongy body'*), is more elastic than the corpus cavernosum and helps to cushion the sensitive vulva. (The vestibular bulbs are homologous to the spongy tissue in the penis through which the urethra passes, and again derive embryologically from the same place.) As we can see, the basic physiology of engorgement and erection is the same for both sexes, with the same tissues and vascular processes occurring in both.

Whilst male engorgement and erection are obvious and deemed essential, the significance of female engorgement and erection are less well-known and understood. So let's explore them further. Two aspects are important to understand: i) pleasure and ii) buffering. As we've seen, engorged, succulent genitals are designed to express our sexual excitement and signal our readiness for penetration. The spongy turgidity of these erectile tissues is essential for our capacity to enjoy the sensations of penetration. Without the cushioning provided by engorgement, the highly sensitive tissues of the vulva press uncomfortably against the hard surfaces of the pubic bone and the internal pelvic outlet, causing pain and possibly abrasions to the soft tissues and skin. So if you're about to have sex without your erectile tissues fully plumped up, it means your body's not ready yet. Take a moment, enjoy some more tantalising and wait till your bulbs and sponges are fully plumped up and juicy before engaging in penetration. Then it can feel wonderful!

Female Arousal

One of the major differences between female and male sexual response is our timing for arousal. You'd never know this from our cultural mythology, especially TV, movies and music videos which depict female sexual response as just like male response, hard and fast. If we want to enjoy our full potential as pleasure divas, we need to understand our female timing, which may be quite different from male sexual response. The number one priority for a woman to surrender to deep sexual pleasure is the down-regulation of her vigilance centre, so she feels safe to shift out of her social brain into deep states of relaxation, interspersed with high states of arousal.[3] In these conditions, a woman can experience extended waves of orgasmic pleasure that continue for hours.

Male readiness for sex is usually an immediate response that begins in the genitals and moves outwards. In contrast, female readiness tends to be more gradual, proceeding from the periphery inwards. Women love to have our bodies caressed and awakened before there's any genital contact because it allows the vigilance centre in our brain to go off duty, so our genitals can swell, open and yield in full responsiveness.

Given that this is the design, it's essential for us to take the initiative and communicate these female needs to our partners, so we teach them what's required and dismantle the cultural mythology. The patriarchal conditioning behind this mythology is that our sexual pleasure depends on our partner. It's *his* responsibility. During sex, this shows up as the critical voice that makes him wrong: he doesn't know what he's doing, sex is more for him than me, he should have done more to turn me on. These unspoken pressures create an agonising double bind for a man and disconnection for both partners.

When we assume authority for a self-referenced sexuality, we take ownership of the delicious sensations in our bodies and genitals, creating our own turn on and asking for what we need to build our pleasure. This unleashes incredible power and energy inside us, so it's not surprising that the cultural mythology has taught us to dumb it down.

Sexuality and Fertility

The vulva also brings us to the connection between sexuality and fertility: desire, arousal and the possible ultimate consequence – a baby! The richness of that connection is often eclipsed by our separation of them as two discrete things. It's true that separating sexuality from fertility can free a woman from the burden of unwanted pregnancies, yet it can also disconnect her from an awareness of her body rhythms and cycles of desire. For example, hormonal contraception (like the Pill, Mirena, Depo Provera and Implanon) can have a dramatic dampening effect on desire, as well as affecting overall health and wellbeing. Despite unlimited opportunity, there may be little desire.

When a woman experiences her natural fertility cycle, she's likely to find her desire directly connected to her fertility. This is hardly surprising considering all the physiological changes occurring in her body around ovulation. As we've seen, her ovaries are busy secreting large amounts of oestrogen, her tubes are positioning themselves ready to capture the released egg, her cervix opens up and releases a clear, glossy mucus to nourish and transport sperm, her uterus pulls higher up into her pelvis and her whole belly is engorged with fluid. Oestrogen adds water, inducing a sensation of plump fullness in the pelvis and breasts.

Oestrogen also causes the vulva to swell markedly around ovulation, creating a succulent fullness in the sensitive tissues, which is amplified by the slippery, wet sensation from cervical mucus as it drizzles down through the vagina and vulva. These sensations feel wonderfully erotic. In addition, oestrogen is a mind-altering substance which, combined with the mid-cycle surge of testosterone, increases libido. This potent mix of physiological and psychological changes primes a woman to be most interested and receptive to the delights of lovemaking around the time of peak fertility. There's often a voluptuous, sensual fulsomeness and openness about her during this time. Of course it's also when she's most likely to conceive, so if she wants to avoid a pregnancy, she can either engage in other forms of lovemaking than penetrative sex or use barrier methods for her fertile days.

Symbolism of the Vulva

Not surprisingly, this exceptional part of our female anatomy is associated with a rich symbolism. Did you know, for example, that universally and from the earliest times, the oyster and marine shellfish were seen as sacred symbols *because of their resemblance to the vulva?* The soft, wet succulence of shellfish is a very obvious physical metaphor for this juicy part of our bodies. This symbolism implies that the vulva itself was venerated as sacred. Historian of religion, Mircea Eliade, noted in his book *Images and Symbols*:

> *"Probably even more than the aquatic origin and the lunar symbolism attaching to oysters and sea-shells, their likeness to the vulva helped to spread belief in their magical virtues."* [4]

In archaeology and anthropology, the shell is found in agrarian, nuptial, initiatory and funeral rites. Long before our culture's shaming of the vulva, the widespread, cross-cultural religious use of shells reflects a heritage in which the sacredness of female genitals was clearly recognised. The shell was seen as an emblem of love, marriage, fertility, fecundity, birth, rebirth into the afterlife, protection from evil and enhancement of wellbeing. [5]

As the site of profound sexual pleasure, the vulva must surely be revered as the sacred domain of the Goddess, if ever there was one in physical form. Its delicate physical beauty and dexterity, it's very female qualities of wetness, succulence and openness, its capacity to render such pleasure to a woman and her partner, epitomise the spirituality of female sexuality. As a portal into orgasmic states, the vulva is also a gateway into spiritual expansion and transcendence. One has only to witness the transformation in the face of a woman after sexual satiation to know that something beatific has been at work!

The exultant spirituality of the vulva is conveyed in the myth of Inanna, the goddess of sexual love. Sylvia Brinton-Perera in her book *Descent to the Goddess*, describes how Inanna celebrates the pleasure, power and beauty of her genitals with total self-love and abandon:

"She calls out to have her body filled, singing praises to her vulva, and bidding Dumuzi come to her bed to 'Plow my vulva, man of my heart.'"[6]

For many women, sexual identity has been based upon external referents and what others need, want or desire. Our culture is full of prescriptions about female sexuality that are completely at odds with our physiology. Making the shift into an inner referenced sexual identity, which derives from our bodies and who we are, is a big journey that's essential for our autonomy. During this transition, we can draw inspiration, courage and strength from the ancient heritage that revered the vulva as sacred and celebrated its power and beauty. Like Inanna, we can take proud ownership of our female genitals, putting the vulva back on the map as sacred site and temple of the divine.

Reflection

What I now know about my vulva that I didn't know before is…

What I most love and appreciate about my vulva is…

When I reflect on this information, what strikes or moves me is…

Affirmation

I cherish my beautiful vulva! It is the Portal of Life and I honour it as a living temple.

Suggestion

If you feel embarrassed about the smell of your genitals, here's my suggestion for overturning your discomfort. Get hold of some pure organic coconut butter (not oil, it's too runny) and each morning before you begin your day, massage a small amount into your vulva. As you move through the day, notice the fragrance of your juices mixed with coconut butter. It's quite a heady mix! The coconut butter seems to both disguise and enhance the natural smell of your vulva and it's a great way to begin to enjoy the aroma. This yummy morning ritual feels wonderful and only takes 30 seconds!

Section Three

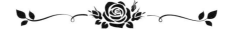

The Blood Mystery

Chapter Nine

❧ ～～～～ ☙

Menstruation

Menstruation is the crowning jewel of this book. I've intentionally saved this chapter till last to give you time to come to a greater appreciation and love for your beautiful female body and all its amazing processes. Now I invite you to extend that same love and appreciation into your bleeding, so you can transform menstrual shame, aversion and secrecy into unshakable pride, poise and self-respect. Not only that. Despite what you've been led to believe, menstruation has the power to connect you to the world of spirit, your soul, and the Earthbody in a really profound way. Let me show you how.

For starters, consider this: menstruation is *"the special blood in which all our lives started"*.[1] If not for the thickening of our mothers' uterine lining, none of us would be here. We each began our lives as a tiny blastocyst burrowing into that rich, red lining, a safe place in which to incubate ourselves into fully formed human beings. Menstruation is thus literally the cradle of life. In some Indigenous and Eastern traditions, menstrual blood is viewed as a participation in the generative power of the female deity and therefore revered as sacred.

Menstruation is a body process that's culturally inscribed with meaning, so the cultural context largely determines how it's viewed. In Western culture, its meaning is overwhelmingly negative and is associated with shame, pollution and the profane. From a young age, we hear menstruation depicted as an embarrassing liability, a kind of 'nose-bleed of the womb'.[2] Like other excretory processes, it's perceived as something distasteful coming from our nether regions. Most women, including health professionals and some feminists, see menstruation as an unfortunate affliction that we'd all be better off without. In the workplace, menses is seen to interfere with productivity and advertising refers to sanitary 'protection' so that 'no-one will ever guess'. The overwhelming message we receive is menstrual suppression and secrecy.[3] It is time we remedied this situation – for ourselves, our daughters and future generations.

Given the pervasiveness of these cultural messages, it's hardly surprising that you'd feel the same way. Menstruation is perhaps the least understood and most maligned of all our female body processes. And yet, I promise you, it's also one of the richest, most powerful and deeply spiritual experiences you can access. Along with the phenomenon of boundary-penetration, which it perfectly exemplifies, it is the quintessential female process; only women bleed without pathology.

The spirituality of menstruation has always been recognised by Native American peoples. If you grew up in the Navajo tradition, your menarche would be seen as an initiation into the power of Changing Woman, the female deity, and it would be celebrated by the whole community.[4] During your menstruating years, you'd be mentored by experienced women, who'd teach you how to exercise the spiritual gifts of menstruation for the benefit of the community. And you'd see the menopausal Elders treated with deep respect, their wisdom highly valued and their authority accepted without question.

Contrast this with Western culture's vacuum around the entire experience of menstruation across the lifespan. We have no rites of passage to initiate girls into their first bleed, so we don't receive the mentoring we need at this formative time. During our menstruating years, we're not taught how to practice the power, magic and transformative potential of our bleeding. And when we reach menopause, we have no idea how to navigate this profound spiritual transition; instead, we're given the message that we're past our 'use-by' date. Given that the 'average' woman spends 2400 days or six consecutive years of her life menstruating,[5] it is shameful that this defining female process and potent spiritual resource remains in the dark.

Menstrual Shame

"It struck me how difficult it is to grow spiritually when for a quarter of your life you're ashamed of who you are." Carla, research participant.

This quote echoes the ample research showing that most Western women begin menstruating from a place of shame. While recent studies indicate more positive experiences for girls at menarche, shame and concealment are very common and are found across cultures. Shame is a toxic, paralysing emotion that impacts our self-worth. Menstrual shame alienates us from our body consciousness, undermining our confidence and trust in ourselves and in our healthy female physiology. Most women have no idea this is the case because it flies under the radar and is widely accepted as 'just how it is'. Menstruation is the Sleeping Beauty who needs rousing from her slumber because the shame and aversion has major individual, social, collective and evolutionary consequences.

One of the key findings from my PhD was that *menstrual shame is a core patriarchal organising principle that instils and perpetuates male dominance and female subordination.* Take a moment to let that sink in. The extent to which we are asleep to this issue is the extent to which we are collaborating with our own subordination and the gender imbalance in our world. Be willing to confront this issue because menstrual shame has implications for future female experiences like birth.

We rarely consider how attitudes to menstruation impact on birth and yet my research clearly showed how menses plays a profound role in shaping women's self-perception, confidence and in/ability to birth fearlessly and powerfully. Because it engenders the perception of female physiology as inherently flawed, menstrual shame is a major factor that predisposes women to approach birth feeling fearful, disempowered and vulnerable to intervention. The alienation from our body which begins at menarche means that many women approach birth disconnected from their sacred, procreative power. What are the consequences of this disconnection?

In the Western world, we have the highest rates of intervention, caesarean surgery and birth trauma we've ever had. Thousands of mothers and babies are missing out on the precious gifts that accompany an undisturbed birth. Because this patriarchal programming is so unconscious, no-one recognises how menstrual shame and aversion bring havoc into the most intimate areas of our lives. When our bleeding is maligned at menarche and derogated during our menstruating years, the sacred potential of menstruation and its contribution to confident birthing is lost. *It does not have to be like this. We have the power to change it.* Naming, understanding and dismantling the toxic pairing of shame and menstruation are critical feminist concerns that we all need to confront.

After the spontaneous blessing of my own menarche, I vowed to always honour menstruation, a vow I've kept to this day. That vow profoundly influenced all my subsequent menstruations, so even when it was painful, messy or embarrassing, I continued to honour my bleed. I knew from personal experience that it was so much more than a physical process. We're going to explore this 'so much more' shortly. Before we do, let's take a look at the physiology of what actually happens when we bleed. Like so many of our female body processes, it is truly mind-blowing!

The Physiology of Menstruation

Did you ever wonder *why* we menstruate? Why the shedding of our womb lining every month? The following description sums it up pretty well:

> *"The endometrium, because of its vital function in sustaining a pregnancy, must be in good condition, and to ensure this, it is completely changed each cycle."*[6]

So simple! A new, glycogen-rich lining is freshly created each month in anticipation of a burrowing embryo – even if that embryo never happens. Photos inside the womb reveal a lush, deep red surface reminiscent of a royal chamber (see colour plates). Many women imagine the inside of their womb as a dark, murky place, so they're usually surprised when I show them a photo of a beautiful red endometrium. So how does it get to be so lush and red? Largely because of its extraordinary blood supply which has some very unusual features. To truly understand the process of menstruation, we need to delve into this remarkable vascular system in some detail.

You'll remember from Chapter Six that the endometrium is comprised of two layers:

1. the **stratum functionalis** (functional layer) which is shed during menses and then regrows

2. the **stratum basalis** (base layer) from which a new functional layer grows at the end of each bleed

Inside the muscular wall of the uterus, the **uterine arteries** branch into several **arcuate arteries** (the arcuate is part of the pelvic bone), which then branch out into **radial arteries** that supply the endometrium. Up to this point, the vascular branching is similar to anywhere else in the body. However once the radial arteries reach the endometrium, an altogether different and completely unique arrangement occurs. (Figure 9.1) Here's what happens. The radial arteries branch again into two different kinds:

1. **straight arteries,** which are short and divide to form capillaries in the stratum basalis

2. **spiral arteries,** which are longer and coil upwards to supply the functional layer, where they form capillaries near the endometrial surface

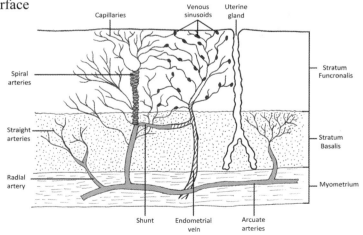

Figure 9.1

Spiral arteries are the key to understanding menstruation. Highly sensitive to the ovarian hormones, they have a unique structure and function seen nowhere else in the body. As the name suggests, the spiral arteries twirl upwards through the growing functional layer in a dense, coiling pattern – a design which ensures a much richer blood supply in the womb lining. Amazingly, this coiling happens because the spiral arteries grow at a much faster rate than the surrounding tissue and as a result, have to continuously compress themselves more tightly into the available space.[7]

A second unique feature of spiral arteries is that they grow little 'shunts' which bypass the capillary network at the endometrial surface and instead connect directly with the veins deep below the surface. Normally arteries end in capillaries in the surface tissue, which is where the veins take over. The 'shunts' are a special adaptation intrinsic to the shedding process, as you'll see.

The brilliance of the design doesn't stop there. Alongside the spiral arteries, there's an extensive network of specially modified veins in the functional layer, with sinuses where the blood pools. These **venous lakes or sinusoids** are thin-walled, allowing large molecules like proteins and blood cells to pass between the blood and surrounding tissues. Blood flows slowly through the venous lakes, allowing it more time to pool and thereby providing a richer nutrient absorption, an ingenious strategy with obvious advantages for a burrowing embryo.

This elaborate network of blood vessels, shunts, glands and venous lakes completely disintegrates during menstruation, along with the entire functional layer. Let's now look at the context in which this happens – the menstrual cycle – and the process of menstruation from beginning to end. It's so much more intelligent, wise and innovative than we ever guessed.

Phases of the Menstrual Cycle

1. **Proliferative Phase:** To proliferate means '*to grow or increase rapidly*' and this perfectly describes what happens in the womb lining after menstruation. In response to hormonal signals from the pituitary and the ovaries, the stratum basalis begins rapidly reconstructing a new

functional layer. Stimulated by rising oestrogen levels, the surface cells heal and regrow, and a whole new vascular network starts to develop. The spiral arteries spring up, growing out to resupply the new functional layer, while the uterine glands enlarge as they begin secreting their juices. In less than a fortnight, the endometrium has completely regrown and progesterone receptors there, primed by oestrogen, are ready to interact with the soon-to-be-released progesterone from the ovulating ovary.

2. **Ovulation:** Once oestrogen levels reach a critical threshold mid-cycle, they drop sharply, triggering a sudden surge of luteinising hormone (LH) from the pituitary gland. This initiates a series of events that culminates in ovulation. First, there's a rapid build-up of fluid in the follicle housing the egg cell, followed by the gradual interruption of the blood flow through the outer follicle wall. As a result, the wall thins and bulges from the ovary surface, before abruptly bursting to propel the egg towards the tube. The LH surge around ovulation also helps transform the ruptured follicle into the **corpus luteum** (hence the name 'luteinising' hormone), which almost immediately begins producing progesterone.

3. **Secretory Phase:** Now the endometrium moves into its secretory phase. In response to rising progesterone levels, the womb lining grows to its thickest. The spiral arteries extend and coil to their maximum, ending in a dense capillary network close to the endometrial surface. Progesterone then transforms the newly grown functional layer into a juicy, succulent lining, from which swollen glands release glycogen into the endometrial surface. Much like what happens in the vulva during arousal, the entire vascular supply and surrounding connective tissue of the endometrium swells with fluid.

The womb lining is now poised at the fullness of its potential: lavish and lush, engorged with spiral arteries and miniature lakes of nutrient-rich blood, this is how it becomes that vibrant red colour. Laden with life-sustaining fluids, the entire endometrial surface is bursting with readiness in anticipation of a blastocyst. If none arrives, what an anticlimax after such an extravagant preparation! About 12 days after ovulation, the corpus luteum in the ovary runs out of progesterone, which means the womb lining loses its hormonal support and prepares to shed.

How this happens is a marvel of biological engineering! The sudden drop in progesterone and oestrogen causes a shrinking of the functional layer so the surface cells begin to die off. As they do, tiny organelles within the cells, known as **lysosomes**, are released. (**Lysosomes** originate in the **Golgi** bodies inside the cells and are full of strong digestive enzymes.) (Figure 9.2) Through this neat little housekeeping gesture, the functional

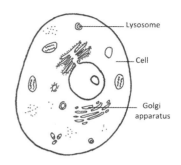

Figure 9.2

layer begins to self-digest in anticipation of the menstrual flow.

This shrinkage also means the spiral arteries have to coil and compress even further, and this in turn, restricts the blood flow to the functional layer. As a result, the spiral arteries begin to kink and buckle and the surrounding tissue starts to die off. Because of the profound constriction in the spiral arteries, most of their blood flow is abruptly redirected through the special 'shunts' into the endometrial veins and sinusoids. With the lining already weakened, this sudden blood redirection creates a rupture of both sinusoids and capillaries, which then spreads throughout the functional layer. The affected area begins to detach and at the same time, the **myometrium** (the smooth muscle layer beneath the stratum basalis) begins to contract rhythmically to assist the shedding process. So much complex, intelligent movement in such a confined space!

4. **Menstrual Phase:** So begins the menstrual phase of the cycle, with bleeding for anywhere between two and seven days. Some women bleed every cycle for four or five days with a good flow on all days. Others have two or three days of heavy bleeding, followed by several days of lighter flow or spotting. Generally, a bright red flow of at least three days indicates healthy fertility. Average blood loss during each period is about 30–40ml, with 80ml considered a heavy loss.

There are huge variations in menstrual characteristics with differences in colour (bright red through to dark brown and everything in between), consistency (watery or thick and clumpy, sometimes with clots), quantity and odour. As you might expect, the qualities of the bleed often reflect the emotional state, stress levels and circumstances of the previous month. There's also enormous diversity in bleeding patterns from cycle to cycle, as well as across the fertile lifespan, with teenagers and peri-menopausal women the most likely to experience heavy bleeds.

Pause for a moment to appreciate the wonder of this design! Through a sophisticated vascular network that completely disintegrates and then regrows each month, the womb lining develops into a luscious surface with all the ingredients to sustain new life. Then, if no blastocyst comes along, the womb elegantly and efficiently breaks down this elaborate construction and releases it. And it does this again and again for decades with no permanent damage. Such a significant disintegration in any other organ would mean serious, even life-threatening consequences. Imagine a similar process in your liver, lungs or stomach. Yet the uterus accomplishes all these complex manoeuvres, often without us being aware of them. The entire process can be pain free. Consider how many times your period has arrived and caught you by surprise. Menstrual pain is not caused by this disintegration in itself and has a different origin which I now describe.

Period Pain or Dysmenorrhoea (*'painful menstrual flow'*)

Debilitating menstrual cramps are not inevitable, nor are they random afflictions. Many people believe it's 'normal' to experience intense pain whilst menstruating, perhaps because many women *do* have that experience, so it *is* normal for them. Yet other women experience no or minimal pain during their bleed. *Excruciating pain during menses is not the design or normal.* Rather, it indicates an imbalance. Let's look for some clues about what that might be.

During menses, the cervical opening needs to dilate to allow the flow out. To a much lesser extent, it's similar to what occurs in labour. As we've already seen, the cervix is an exquisitely sensitive, responsive part of our womb and our sexuality, with a strong energetic connection to the heart. So we'd expect to feel some sensations during its opening at menstruation and these sensations are meant to be within our capacity to handle, with the appropriate care and love.

In my birth preparation sessions, I tell my clients that the cervix has ears – she hears every word you say! Because she's a sphincter, she needs to feel safe and responds best to loving, kind and appreciative words.[8] If a labouring woman's partner whispers 'sweet nothings' in her ear during labour, she'll literally feel her cervix soften and open. The same thing applies during menses. Our cervix needs to feel safe and cared for, and to hear loving, kind and appreciative words from us; then she'll respond in kind.

The physiological basis of intense pain during menstruation is an *overproduction of prostaglandins*. You may remember from Chapter Six that prostaglandins are chemical messengers that act locally like hormones. Produced in different tissues all over the body in both sexes, prostaglandins are part of our body's capacity to deal with injury by regulating blood flow, inflammation and the formation of clots. They're also involved in the contraction and relaxation of the gut muscles and the airways, so they do lots of useful things. Only two in particular, **PGE_2** and **PGF_{2a}**, are associated with menstrual cramping.

Progesterone inhibits prostaglandin release, so when progesterone levels drop at the end of the cycle, prostaglandin production increases – for some women excessively. Both the constriction of the spiral arteries and contractions of the smooth uterine muscle are mediated by prostaglandins in the endometrium, so an overproduction leads to excessive contractions, not unlike those of early labour. At high levels, prostaglandins produce inflammation, not just in the uterus but in other parts of the body, inducing painful symptoms like nausea, vomiting, diarrhoea, sweating, fever and distress. Medically this is called **primary dysmenorrhoea**, whereas **secondary dysmenorrhoea** is pain associated with conditions like endometriosis, fibroids or infection.

No-one really knows why some women make more prostaglandins than others. For some, it may be a genetic predisposition, their mothers or other female relatives having had the same experience. However, while genes may give rise to a tendency towards certain conditions, they are not necessarily our destiny. We now know that we can permanently alter our genes' behaviour through epigenetics and we also know that the genes are switched on by what's happening in the cell membrane.[9]

So we need to consider the environment in which the cells are marinating, especially our diet, stress levels and subconscious beliefs. These three factors are known contributors to excessive prostaglandin production. If you suffer with dysmenorrhoea, then please know that it's entirely possible to permanently eliminate excruciating pain as a routine way of menstruating. My e-book, *Befriending Your Bleed* (available from www.sharonmoloney.com) is a map for how to do this.

Premenstrual Sensitivity (PMS aka Premenstrual Syndrome)

PMS or premenstrual syndrome is the medical term for a range of physical and emotional symptoms leading up to menstruation, including bloating, fatigue, breast tenderness, headaches, anger, depression, irritability and social withdrawal. These cyclic changes require greater self-care, understanding and down-time. The discrepancy between these needs and the demands of a linear workplace make the 'diagnosis' of PMS a kind of pressure-relieving valve between the two.[10] While the inclusion of premenstrual dysphoric disorder (PMDD) in the *DSM–5*[11] gave women diagnostic legitimacy for time off work, it further pathologised premenstrual sensitivity. I have a completely different take on this phenomenon, so let me share it with you.

Out of 11 symptoms listed in the *DSM–5*, only one includes the physical manifestations; the other ten are emotional/behavioural. These same emotional/behavioural experiences can be understood as a naturally heightened **premenstrual sensitivity,** which is difficult to manage in our culture because our legitimate needs are not being met. Although it's treated as a medical disorder, premenstrual sensitivity is potentially one of menstruation's greatest gifts. Despite what many people believe, the sensitivity is not the result of 'raging hormones'; it's actually the opposite.

The heightened sensitivity of the premenstruum is a consequence of the *hormonal withdrawal* that triggers bleeding. For centuries, Indigenous peoples have highly valued this state as one of greater spiritual permeability and their seclusion practices enabled women to maximise their receptivity to Spirit. So let's now look at the hormonal state behind premenstrual sensitivity to better understand what's going on.

During the menstrual cycle, the ovaries release first oestrogen and then after ovulation, progesterone into our blood stream. Oestrogen is relationship oriented, improves cognition, stabilises mood and generates a sense of wellbeing. Progesterone has a slightly sedative effect (it can act as a surgical anaesthetic in very high doses), so it tends to dampen libido and dull perception. [12] Hormones are powerful mind-altering substances and oestrogen in particular predisposes us to minimise unpalatable truths in order to maintain relationships and accommodate others' needs. So when oestrogen and progesterone levels plummet before the bleed, the buffer they provide is no longer there. Instead we have sharper clarity of perception and are much more likely to call it when the emperor wears no clothes!

However, this naturally occurring sensitivity can also be adversely impacted by hormonal imbalances that make it more inflammatory and difficult to manage. For some women (and for many women some of the time), premenstrual sensitivity is a testing time that requires greater awareness, self-control and self-care, less stimulation and more seclusion. Oestrogen dominance is the main culprit, not surprising given that our environment and food chain are overloaded with chemical substances that mimic oestrogen.

Xenoestrogens, as they are called, are present in pesticides which contaminate our food, plastics like the packaged fast food meals designed for the microwave, clingwrap, plastic bottles and containers, industrial compounds like dioxin, and non-biodegradable industrial contaminants. Millions of tons of these substances have found their way into our food supply and our homes.

In addition, the animals we eat are hormone fed. Chickens are given synthetic oestrogen to make their chests bigger and red meat animals are also given hormone-containing feed to spur their growth and increase profits. When we eat these animal products, we absorb the xenoestrogens, which interfere with the normal receptor response to our own endogenous oestrogen. A main side effect of excess oestrogen is fluid retention; oestrogen binds salt, which in turn binds water. In addition to sore breasts, bloating and weight gain, this creates swelling and irritation of the brain membrane, causing headaches, dizziness and irritability. Reducing salt helps alleviate fluid retention and minimising exposure to environmental pollutants and plastics, eating organic foods and filtering water are all ways of avoiding xenoestrogens.

PMS as Spiritual Imbalance

In the Introduction to this book, I spoke about women adapting to the workplace by adopting a masculine psychology and how damaging this is for our health, fertility and spirituality. Native American elder, Paula Gunn Allen, points out:

"One of the biggest mistakes modern women make – and it's because they have been coerced into it – is that they keep using male models of spirituality... all of these models are about how men integrate their immortal self with their mortal self. Men have a different physiology and their methods are designed to work for that physiology, not for the physiology of women." [13]

As we've seen repeatedly in this book, female physiology is rich, unique, and completely unlike male physiology, so we need ways of staying in balance and connected to our spirituality that are appropriate to us. Ignoring our physiology and acting just like men messes with our nervous and endocrine systems. Paula Gunn Allen maintains PMS is a spiritual condition, not a medical condition, and that it's our intelligent body's way of saying: 'Hey, listen! Something's not right here'. The following true story illuminates this point well.

Lynne began menstruating at age 11 and for the next 20 years experienced heavy bleeding and chronic PMS that made her suicidally depressed. She developed ovarian cysts and breast lumps, and when she became pregnant, vomited for the entire nine months. Anything to do with being female brought her pain. Eventually Lynne began looking within herself for answers:

"Sitting quietly one day, I asked myself why an otherwise healthy person (I rarely had a cold or complaint of any description) should be plagued only with these womanly problems. The answer came loud and clear – guilt! "Guilt about what?" I asked this mysterious voice. It answered: "Everything that represents the woman in you gives rise to feelings of shame." I almost wept with the revelation." [14]

The origins of Lynne's guilt lay in her early family environment, which was one of sexual repression, in which she felt "programmed to reject all the parts of me that spelled 'woman'". Her first bleed was an occasion of humiliation, secrecy and shame, in which she'd imbued both her mother's fear and her father's disgust.

As Lynne attended to her inner voice, it guided her to accept and love her femaleness. She soaked in perfumed baths, had her hair restyled and bought some makeup, lingerie and clothes that accentuated her femininity. As Lynne learned to welcome her monthly flow, for the first time in 20 years, she experienced trouble-free periods. No PMS, no cramps, no flooding. The change was dramatic and enduring; the guilt, shame and negativity of the past dissolved. Her menstruation reflected the love and care she gave to herself, and her femaleness became the source of her self-esteem and empowerment.

Lynne's story shows what's possible for any woman who wants to transform menstrual shame into a loving relationship with her femaleness.

The Symbolism of Menstruation

In cultures around the world, menstruation has been associated with a range of symbols. In her ground-breaking book, *Her Blood is Gold*, Lara Owen identified four archetypal symbols of menses: the moon, the blood, the Earth and the snake. [15] Before the advent of artificial light, the menstrual cycle was synchronised with the phases of the **moon**, so women ovulated at full moon and menstruated during the new moon, a synchrony that connected us intrinsically with the greater processes of Nature. For us as mammals, **blood** is life itself. Normally, blood circulates *inside* the body, its external appearance signifying injury, disease, even death. Menstrual blood is unique because it is healthy, life-giving and nonpathological. The **Earth** is the macrocosm of which we are the microcosm. As our fertile planet creates life abundantly, we also create life inside our female bodies. The ancient emblem of transformation, the **snake**, sheds its skin regularly, just as we shed our womb lining. Snake represents the cycle of death and rebirth in which we expand into the more of who we are.

These archetypes, which originated with the pre-patriarchal female deity, the Goddess, continue as living symbols inside our bodies. Accessing their energies can enable us to penetrate the cultural denigration of the female body and connect with its spiritual potency. Keep them in mind as you go about your daily life and you'll be surprised by how often they appear as reminders of your menstruation and its connection to the sacred.

Female Origins of the Menstrual Taboo

The word 'taboo' derives from the Polynesian *tapua*, which means both 'sacred' and 'menstruation'. [16] A taboo evokes elements of dread and awe, of something so frightening, sacred and powerful that it must be set apart. The perception of menstruation as sacred and powerful, and therefore needing to be separated from ordinary life, was implicit in the development of the earliest menstrual taboos. A compelling body of archaeological evidence from ancient pre-patriarchal times shows that the first deity was female and that women's bodies were honoured, as was menstruation. Hundreds of female figurines emphasising bellies, breasts, vulva and buttocks, and widespread use of red ochre as a menstrual symbol, reveal that our earliest forbears endowed both the female body and menstruation with sacred, miraculous powers. [17]

With the beginnings of patriarchy about 5000 years ago, the Goddess, who had been worshipped for some 30,000 years, was reduced to the status of a lewd, depraved figure and in her place, a male deity was imposed. [18] The social consequence of this deposition was the replacement of the sacred associations of the female body and menstruation with shame, pollution and the profane. Not surprisingly, Western anthropologists schooled in a patriarchal mindset assumed that menstrual taboos were simply a form of female subordination. While this is certainly the case in some cultural contexts, other cultures preserved the veneration of the female deity and the female body, including menstruation.

Anthropologists Thomas Buckley and Alma Gottlieb describe various studies on Indigenous societies, where menstruation is conceptualised as a spiritual phenomenon:

"Many menstrual taboos, rather than protecting society from a universally ascribed feminine evil, explicitly protect the perceived creative spirituality of menstruous women from the influence of others in a more neutral state, as well as protecting the latter in turn from the potent, positive spiritual force ascribed to such women." [19]

In these Indigenous societies, a range of menstrual practices enable women to exercise autonomy, authority and social influence, rather than subordinating them to men. These traditions are inspiring because they're a faithful remnant that's carried the flame down the ages to hand on to us.

The Spiritual Power of Menstruation

Paradoxical as it may seem, *menstruation signifies female spiritual power*. Whilst this deep truth has been hidden from us in Western patriarchal culture, Indigenous peoples like the Native Americans have preserved practices that cultivate the spiritual power of menstruation. Yurok women, for example, retreated to the Moon Lodge while menstruating to honour the life-sustaining power of their blood, strengthen their connection with

Earth, and open themselves to Spirit.[20] From a young age, women were taught how to exercise the spiritual gifts of menstruation for healing self and others; these gifts included creative problem-solving, spiritual insight and guidance for the wider community.

Native American elder, Brooke Medicine Eagle, teaches that the function of menstruation is to 'call for vision', not just for ourselves, but for our family, our community, and our world.[21] I imagine women in the Moon Lodge serving as spiritual ambassadors by taking their community concerns to Spirit. I imagine them sharing amongst themselves matters like: this little boy seems unbalanced, so what might be helpful for him? Or, that woman can't get pregnant – what does she need? Or the community is grappling with this particular issue – how can we best resolve it? I imagine answers to these questions coming from Spirit into the receptivity of the women's wombs, so that their bleeding made a vital contribution to the community.

In our Western cultural vacuum around menstruation, it's difficult to imagine the purpose, fulfilment, authority and power these practices would give to individual women and to women as a group. When we contrast this approach with our history of secrecy and contempt, it's easy to see how menstrual shame and disdain have divested us of our spiritual power. This perspective throws a different light on experiences like PMS, prostaglandin overproduction, painful periods or heavy bleeding.

Our beautiful female bodies express their grievances so eloquently. As Penelope Shuttle and Peter Redgrove observed, menstruation has been *"despised, tabooed, neglected, and ... as if in response to this spiteful treatment, in many women hurts."*[22] Mistreatment of menstruation is like short-circuiting an electrical current and then wondering why fuses blow and sparks fly! When the spiritual energy of menstruation is tied up in knots, its power gets turned back on itself painfully.

It's entirely possible to transform menstrual pain, shame and aversion into the spiritual practice of menstruation as a source of power, authority and loving connection to Earth. If every woman made the commitment to self-love as Lynne did earlier in this chapter, the cumulative effect would change our world dramatically. Just for a moment, imagine what life would look like if we, as a society, honoured women's bodies and menstruation as sacred. Imagine a social norm where women took the time to care for themselves whilst menstruating and bled with dignity. Imagine if we learned as a collective to practice the spiritual gifts of our bleeding and developed the skills to access its visions, clear-sighted problem-solving, intuitive wisdom, guidance and connection to Spirit. Those gifts, which are uniquely ours as female, endow us with a specific kind of biological leadership. And the world urgently needs us to exercise that leadership – NOW!

Reflection

What I now know about menstruation that I didn't know before is…

What I most love and appreciate about my bleed is…

When I reflect on this information, what strikes or moves me is…

Affirmation

Menstruation is beautiful, powerful and sacred. It fills me with power and beauty.

Suggestion

Next time you menstruate, wear some cloth pads so you can see, smell and feel your menstrual flow. Soak the pads in a bucket of water and then give the soak water to a plant that needs some extra nourishment. Be aware of the plant's gratitude as you pour the water into its roots and pray a blessing to connect you to Earth.

Conclusion

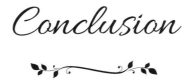

Now that we've reached the end of our journey together, it's time for me to pass the baton over to you. You now know the incredible riches inside your body – the soft sweetness, the juiciness, the intelligence and resourcefulness, the creativity, the sheer strength and raw power, and the profound spirituality. It all belongs to you, to deploy at your will, in whatever way you choose. So now I have an invitation for you.

In the Introduction, I spoke about a reciprocally rewarding relationship between the Earthbody and our female body. As you know, our womb holds the capacity to resonate with Earth's womb, the energetic force field of the magma core. This cosmological power is something *we* possess that men do not. It's our gift. Our intimate connection to Earth and to the Divine Matrix means we can grow new life inside us *and* we can also catalyse cultural change in ways that men cannot. Men can participate in this cosmic potential through ceremony, through heart-opening connection and through lovemaking, so our work also involves creating co-empowered, respectful relationships with men, who have their own contribution to make. We all know that significant change is urgently needed if we are to create a sustainable future, not only for ourselves but for all the other life-forms on the Planet.

When the first photos of the Earth taken from space beamed back the image of our beautiful blue orb suspended against a black backdrop, something profound shifted in human consciousness. At the same time, powerful electron microscopes were penetrating the subatomic world of inner space with images that challenged previous notions of solid matter. Ethicist Meredith Michaels observed that the language of space exploration and human embryology inevitably collided.[1] Outer space and inner space are mirrors of each other. From its original Enlightenment beginnings, science began to show us the indeterminacy of the Universe at the subatomic level or put another way, "*a fundamental ontological openness in the world itself.* "[2] What does that mean for you and me?

What it means is that our human consciousness co-creates and participates in the unfolding Universe *in ways that change it*. That is a truly sober, awe-filled notion, so pause for a moment and let it sink in. For two million years, humans evolved within *"a matrix woven equally of nature and culture.* "[3] During this time, our cultural effects did not have the capacity to fundamentally alter Earth's macrocosm. That is no longer the case. As our population has exploded and we've become more and more alienated from nature, our cultural impacts have now irrevocably altered many of the major life-support systems of our Planet. Climate change, nuclear accidents and environmental degradation are escalating imperatives we urgently need to address.

More than ever before, our FEMALE mother-bear ferocity and our biological leadership are needed to ensure that Earth becomes our top priority. Earth is our Mother, a living, breathing, conscious Being, who's communicating with us clearly. She has a raging fever! Current changes in ocean surface temperature, rainfall and sea levels are irreversible for more than 1000 years after CO_2 emissions are completely stopped! And we're nowhere near that. Earth now needs an army of female warriors to be her voice, her arms and legs, her ambassadors. How can you participate in this pivotal moment?

Here's my invitation: be willing to transform your relationship with your body, to respect it as sacred and to act out of that knowledge. When you love your beautiful female body, you can teach others how to do that too. And as you practice genuine self-respect, you will be guided about what's yours to do. Earth will support you with profound gratitude. If you ask her, Earth will inspire you with practical ways to make *your* contribution. Each of us has a small piece of the solution and that small piece matters enormously. This is how we can powerfully accelerate the cultural transformation needed to move us towards sustainable sanity.

Deep down, we are fearful about what's happening in our world, wondering how to make a difference, or even if it's too late. Reclaiming the sacredness of our female bodies is a very personal way we can remedy our alienation from Nature and re-establish our intimate connection with Earth.

Why is this so important? It's crucial because research shows that in places where the female body is honoured, the Earthbody is also honoured. When enough of us do that – women are 50% of the world's population – it has the power to transform the morphogenetic field in which we live, so that the creativity, inspiration and innovative solutions we need are unleashed.

We have a secret in our culture. It is that women are STRONG and POWERFUL! When we act together in solidarity with one another, with our menfolk and with Earth, we can create what's needed for our planetary survival and our thriving. It is *our time* now to take the reins and guide our families, communities, governments and world into that sustainable future. And you can't rise to that occasion unless you love yourself and activate your female power first. So my parting words to you are: *love your beautiful female body, it is sacred; love your bleeding, it is powerful.* Welcome your amazing female power with open arms, loving heart and receptive womb, and see what happens. Miracles will follow!

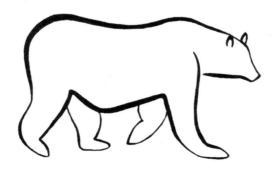

Reflection

What I now know about being female on Planet Earth that I didn't know before is…

What I most love and appreciate about being female on Planet Earth is…

When I reflect on this information, what strikes or moves me is…

Affirmation

My body and Earth's body are one; my womb resonates in perfect harmony with Earth's magma force field.

Suggestion

i) Download the MP3 recording, *Activate Your Female Power,* available from the website and listen to it daily for 28 days. It will support you to consolidate the changes generated by this book.

ii) Spend regular time on your own in Nature with your bare feet on the ground –in your backyard, sitting under a tree, beside a creek or river, on a beach, in a rainforest or a desert. Open your heart and speak to Earth as if She hears every word you're saying; then wait and listen for Her response.

iii) Lie down on your belly on the ground, close your eyes and let your whole body attune to Earth's heartbeat. Ask Her to bring your womb into perfect alignment with Her womb. Want that to happen, allow it to happen, and welcome it into your body.

About the Author

Sharon Moloney

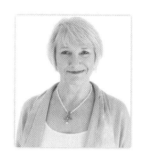

Sharon is an author, childbirth educator, fertility therapist, supporter of midwives and clinical hypnotherapist specialising in women's health. She has always been fascinated by spirituality, Nature and the female body. Ever since her first menstruation, which was a spontaneous spiritual awakening, she has loved being female. A conversion experience in early adulthood led Sharon to join a contemplative monastery and although she loved the silence, meditation and prayer, she felt spiritually disembodied. Having fallen ill, she left the monastery three years later.

When she decided to have her second child, she encountered fertility problems that medication could not help. As a result, she began an in-depth study of female anatomy and physiology with the goal of figuring out how to regain her fertility and health. In the process, she discovered her 'path with heart,' and realised she had been looking for 'God' in all the wrong places. Sacredness was right here, under her nose, all along! She decided to dedicate the rest of her life to sharing this mind-altering information with other people. Her health recovered and at the age of 40, Sharon was overjoyed to be pregnant and give birth to her daughter.

From this time on, she began training in women's health focussing on fertility, pregnancy, childbirth, counselling and hypnotherapy. After completing a writing diploma, Sharon deepened her knowledge of women's health with a Master's of Women's Studies, specialising in menstruation, birth and women's spirituality. Concerned at the lack of research into the spiritual dimensions of these core female experiences, she went on to gain her PhD, exploring both menstruation and birth as spiritual phenomena. She disseminated her research findings nationally and internationally through peer-reviewed journal articles, book chapters, articles in midwifery journals and other publications. In the process, she became a passionate ambassador for the sacredness of the female body, and a spokesperson for the intimate relationship between the female body and the Earthbody.

Sharon has worked at the tertiary level as tutor, guest lecturer, mentor and research assistant. For eight years, she served as a counsellor with a dedicated pregnancy counselling agency, and in 2004, she established a holistic reproductive health program in North Queensland, training counselling staff in fertility, contraception, pregnancy, birth, and reproductive loss. She spent five years as a consumer reviewer for the Midwifery Peer Review Program run by the Australian College of Midwives, a role which inspired her dedication to supporting midwives. Her private practice as a women's health educator, counsellor, hypnotherapist and female ambassador is informed by the depth of her extensive studies, professional work and personal experience.

Sharon loves being female, dancing, travelling, cooking, martial arts, studying spirituality, spending time in Nature, and enjoying fun times with friends. She is the author of *Activate Your Female Power* and lives beside a beautiful river on the Gold Coast, Queensland, with her family, which includes a cat and a dog. You can contact her at: www.sharonmoloney.com

Recommended Resources

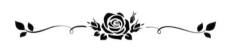

Dr Sharon Moloney

Miraculous Moments

Sharon Moloney knows that being female is both a privilege and a challenge in a male-oriented world. So she created the sacred space of *Miraculous Moments* to support you to navigate those challenges with savvy intelligence, humour and grace. *Miraculous Moments* is a consciously maintained energy field, dedicated to restoring the sacredness of the female body and the beauty of its reproductive power. Inside this secure container, the invisible energies underpinning the visible world are seen as the primary reality and enlisted to facilitate your healing, autonomy and manifesting. When you step through this portal, Grace is waiting. And with Grace on your side, miracles can happen!

Miraculous Moments **provides:**

- **Fertility therapy** to identify and uproot subconscious barriers to conception and replace them with a positive attraction that draws the spirit of the baby to you; support for IVF so that your body is flooded with endorphins to create a blissful landing pad for your embryo.

- **Menstrual consciousness education** to transform your relationship with your cycle, eliminate shame and access the deep spirituality of menstruation, so it turns you into a woman of power; hypnosis to reprogram your attitudes and relieve menstrual pain.

- **Birth preparation** to dismantle fear and align with the natural laws that govern the process, so you can give birth from your centre of power; support for necessary caesarean birth so you can still retain your power and create the best experience possible.

- **Hypnotherapy** to resolve and transform birth trauma; to come to peace with a miscarriage/stillbirth/neonatal death/termination by connecting with the spirit of the baby; to support you through reproductive surgeries with your power intact.

- **Support for Midwives** to unburden workplace constraints; to debrief from vicarious birth trauma and stillbirth/neonatal deaths; to relieve stress and create sustainable practice strategies.

- **Workshops and Training** on the spiritual dimensions of fertility, menstruation, pregnancy, birth and midwifery; grief and loss in maternity care; women's biological leadership attributes.

- **E-books, MP3 recordings and on-line courses** are available from www.sharonmoloney.com

Environment

TreeSisters

Imagine a reforestation revolution ignited by the shared creativity and courage of a global network of millions of women. TreeSisters is a non-profit organisation aiming to radically accelerate tropical reforestation by engaging the unique feminine consciousness, gifts and leadership of women everywhere and focusing it towards global action. TreeSisters are planting over a million trees a year, and they are now calling for women to plant a billion trees a year, by becoming a treesister and contributing monthly to tropical reforestation.

www.treesisters.org

Women's Environmental Network

WEN's mission is to make the connections between women's health and well-being and an environmentally sustainable future.

www.wen.org.uk

Fertility

A comprehensive resource for all fertility matters is **Natural Fertility Info.**

http://natural-fertility-info.com

Menstruation

Lara Owen is a writer and researcher whose work explores the public/private interface of menstrual experience. As a consultant, she helps progressive, female-friendly workplaces develop practical, supportive policies. She is the author of "Her Blood Is Gold: Awakening to the Wisdom of Menstruation" and has been an advocate for menstrual awareness and wellbeing for over 25 years. For more information and to get in touch, please visit:

http://laraowen.com

JuJu Menstrual Cups – If a woman menstruates from the age of 13 until the age of 50, she will have 400 cycles over a period of 37 years and will use 10,500 tampons or pads over her lifetime. JuJu cup will save you thousands of dollars and reduce your eco footprint.

www.juju.com.au

Spiritual Psychotherapy

Kaye Gersch, PhD has a deep understanding of the human condition, including women's spirituality from a feminist perspective. Her professional work spans Jungian psychotherapy, dream work, clinical supervision, couples therapy, lecturing and writing. Although her journey has been filled with detours and false turns, she has learned to trust that some overarching wisdom corrects her path. Dr Gersch is forever curious about life and has a perpetual love of learning. She convenes an online Jung Study Group and offers workshops of many kinds.

www.kayegersch.com
E: womenspirituality@gmail.com
Ph: +61 (0)438 221 334 (Aus)

Sexuality

Layla Martin - Sexuality both fascinated and scared Layla Martin from a very young age and she's always been obsessed with it. She studied human sexuality at Stanford and then spent the next 10 years in the jungles of Asia working with Tantric masters. Layla now blends ancient Tantric wisdom with modern science to help detox people's unhealthy relationships with sex. Her YouTube channel has more than 45 million views, Cosmopolitan calls her a 'sexpert extraordinaire' and Women's Health Magazine has dubbed her the 'headmistress of pleasure'.

https://www.layla-martin.com/
https://www.youtube.com/laylamartintv

Alex Fox expresses a delightful mix of professionalism and playfulness as an Australian based sensuality specialist and certified sexological bodyworker. Her passion is creating embodiment retreats, workshops, and online sessions which support individual awareness for collective growth. Alex works internationally with adults from all sexes, genders, identities, and abilities who desire to increase sexual confidence, including intimate relating skills.

www.alexfox.com.au
E: info@alexfox.com.au

Shamanic De-armoring is a deep healing process that utilizes pleasure to transform cellular pain tapes held within the body. As you release your armor, pain and numbness, you discover how your life force energy has the power to transform and heal. You come home to yourself and your own essence. Your sexual-soul life force energy starts pulsing through your body with greater power and magnitude. You embrace your true nature and set yourself free.

"We are much more than we have even imagined ourselves to be."

www.shamanicdearmoring.com
E: info@shamanicdearmoring.com

References

References

The original anatomy and physiology information for this book was derived from:

- L. Bostock, S. Luck & S. Merrell, 1989, *The Human Body,* Galley Press.

- Elaine Marieb & Jon Mallatt, 1992, *Human Anatomy,* The Benjamin/Cummings Publishing Company.

- G. J. Tortora & S. R. Grabowski, 1993, *Principles of Anatomy and Physiology,* Harper Collins College Publishing.

- A. Vander, J. Sherman & D. Luciano, 1990, *Human Physiology,* McGraw-Hill Publishing.

- David Williams (Ed.), 1987, *The Way Your Body Works,* Artists House Publishing.

- Kathleen Wilson, 1988, *Anatomy and Physiology: in Health and Illness,* Churchill Livingston.

More recent general anatomy and physiology information came from:

- Elaine Marieb, PhD, 2014, *Human Anatomy and Physiology,* 9th Ed. Pearson.

Introduction

1. I have described my experience of menarche in my e-book: *Mothers and Daughters: Preparing for Menstruation*, available from my website: www.sharonmoloney.com

2. Jo Murphy-Lawless, 1998, *Reading Birth and Death.* Cork: Cork University Press, p. 261–62.

3. Charlene Spretnak, 1991, *States of Grace: The recovery of meaning in the postmodern age*. San Francisco: Harper.

4. If you regularly listen to the recording that accompanies this book (freely available from the website www.ActivateYourFemalePower. com) it will teach you how to access your deep relaxation response.

5. Patrick Hanks (Ed.), 1979, *Collins English Dictionary*, Australian Edition.

6. Colin Tipping, 2000, *Radical Forgiveness*, Gateway, Gill and MacMillan, p. 27.

7. Penny Lewis, 2002, *Integrative Holistic Health, Healing and Transformation: A guide for practitioners, consultants and administrators*. Springfield: Charles C. Thomas Publisher.

8. Tipping, op. cit. p. 29.

9. Caroline Myss, 1997, *Anatomy of the Spirit*. Sydney: Bantam Books, p. 40.

10. *Collins English Dictionary*, op. cit.

11. Werner Heisenberg, 1989, *Physics and Philosophy*. London: Penguin.

12. David Bohm, 1980, *Wholeness and the Implicate Order*. London: Ark.

13. Fritjof Capra, 2000, *The Tao of Physics: An exploration of the parallels between modern physics and Eastern mysticism*, 4th Ed. Boston: Shambhala Publications.

14. Sylvia Brinton-Perera, 1981, *Descent to the Goddess*, Toronto: Inner City Books, p. 13.

15. Sallie McFague, 1987, *Models of God*, Philadelphia: Fortress Press, p. 113.

16. Peggy Reeves Sanday, 1981, *Female Power and Male Dominance: On the origins of sexual inequality*, Cambridge University Press.

Chapter One

1. Jaap van der Wal, 2010, *Embryo in Motion*, DVD, Portland Branch of the Anthroposophical Society of America.

2. Ibid.

3. Ibid.

4. The Holy Bible, Revised Standard Version, Catholic Edition for India, 1973, Collins.

5. Irene Elia, 1989, *The Female Animal*, Henry Holt & Company, p. 158/9.

6. Ibid. p. 160.

7. Pamela Hill Nettleton, 2015, "Brave Sperm and Demure Eggs: Fallopian Gender Politics on YouTube", *Feminist Formations*, 27, (1): 24-45, John Hopkins University Press.

8. Daniella Zuccarello, Alberto Ferlin, Andrea Garolla, Massimo Menegazzo, Lisa Perilli, Guido Ambrosini, and Carlo Foresta, 2011, "How the Human Spermatozoa Sense the Oocyte: A New Role of SDF1-CXCR4 Signalling." *International Journal of Andrology*, 34 (6, 2): 554–65.

9. Jaap van der Wal, op. cit.

Chapter Two

1. Jaap van der Wal, op. cit.

2. Elaine Marieb, 2014, op. cit.

3. Ibid.

4. Emily Nagoski, 2015, *Come as You Are*, N.Y: Simon and Schuster Paperbacks.

5. Elaine Marieb, op. cit.

6. Irene Elia, op cit., p. 164

7. Lesley Rogers, 2002, *Sexing the Brain*, Columbia University Press, p. 31.

8. National Geographic: *Special Issue – The Shifting Landscape of Gender. Gender Revolution*, January, 2017, Vol. 231, No.1, Official Journal of the National Geographic Society.

Chapter Three

1. Deepak Chopra, 2009, *Reinventing the Body, Resurrecting the Soul*, Potter/Ten Speed Harmony.

2. Werner Heisenberg, op. cit.

3. David Bohm, op. cit.

4. Joseph Chilton Pearce, 1992, *Evolution's End: Claiming the potential of our intelligence.* San Francisco: Harper.

5. Candace Pert, 1997, *Molecules of Emotion: The science behind mind-body medicine.* New York: Touchstone.

6. Bohm, op. cit.

7. Karl Pribram, 1998, The holographic brain. In *Thinking Allowed: Conversations on the leading edge of knowledge and discovery*, with Dr Jeffrey Mishlove. http://homepages.ihug.co.nz/~sai/pribram.htm. Retrieved 23 June, 2008.

8. Other determinants of health include genetic, social, cultural and environmental factors. My focus is on personal determinants.

Chapter Four

1. A. Domar, K. Rooney, B. Wiegand, E. Orav, M. Alper, B. Bergen, & J. Nikolovski, 2011. "Impact of a group mind/body intervention on pregnancy rates in IVF patients." *Fertility and Sterility, 95, 7, June.*

2. Irene Elia, op. cit. p. 4.

3. Ibid. p. 4.

4. Joan Borysenko, PhD, 1996. *A Woman's Book of Life*, Riverhead Books, Berkley Publishing Group.

5. Ibid. p. 15.

6. Irene Elia, op. cit, p. 4.

7. Ibid. p. 17.

8. Sheila Kitzinger, 1983, *Women's Experience of Sex*, Collins, p. 48.

9. Clarissa Pinkola Estes, 1993, *Women Who Run With the Wolves*, Random House, p. 33.

Chapter Five

1. Geraldine Lux Flanagan, 1996, *Beginning Life*, Doubleday, p. 27.

2. Niels Lauersen and Colette Bouchez, 1991, *Getting Pregnant*, Ballantine Books, p. 8.

3. Amy Thurmond, M.D., 2008, "Fallopian Tube Catheterization", *Seminars in Interventional Radiology*, 2008, 25 (4): 425–431.

4. J. Bouyer, J. Coste, and T. Shojaei, 2003, "Risk factors for Ectopic Pregnancy: A Comprehensive Analysis Based on a Large Case-Control, Population-based study in France", *American Journal of Epidemiology*, 157 (3): 185–194.

Chapter Six

1. Sheila Kitzinger, op, cit, p. 46.

2. Federation of Feminist Women's Health Centers, 1991, *A New View of a Woman's Body*, Feminist Press, p. 69.

3. Evelyn L. Billings, John J. Billings and Maurice Catarinich, 1989, *Billings Atlas of the Ovulation Method: the mucus patterns of fertility and infertility*, Ovulation Method Research and Reference Centre of Australia.

4. Erik Odeblad, 1994, "The Discovery of Different Types of Cervical Mucus and the Billings Ovulation Method", *The Bulletin of the Ovulation Method Research and Reference Centre of Australia*, 21, 3, pp 3-35.

5. Ibid, p. 14.

6. Eileen and Isidore Gersh, 1981, *The Biology of Women*, Junction Books, p. 198.

7. Sarah Buckley, 2015, *Hormonal Physiology of Childbearing: Evidence and Implications for Women, Babies, and Maternity Care*, Childbirth Connection Programs, National Partnership for Women and Families.

8. Sarah Buckley, 2005, Undisturbed Birth: Nature's blueprint for ease and ecstasy. *Journal of Prenatal and Perinatal Psychology and Health*, 17(4): 261–288.

9. Sheri Winston, 2010, *Women's Anatomy of Arousal*, Mango Garden Press, p. 67.

10. Jamie Sams, in Bonnie Horrigan (Ed.), 1996, *Red Moon Passage*, Thorsons, p.172–3.

11. Gregg Braden, 2007, *The Divine Matrix: Bridging time, space, miracles and belief*, Carlsbad, California: Hay House.

Chapter Seven

1. Anna Knöfel Magnusson, 2009, *Vaginal Corona: Myths surrounding virginity*, RFSU (Swedish Association for Sexuality Education).

2. Larry Lipshultz, Alexander Pastuszak, Andrew Goldstein, Annamaria Giraldi, Michael Perelman, 2016, *Management of Sexual Dysfunction in Men and Women: An Interdisciplinary Approach*, Springer.

3. Sheila Kitzinger, op. cit. p. 38.

4. Ibid, p. 48.

5. Alice Kahn Ladas, Beverly Whipple and John Perry, 1982, *The G Spot*, Dell Publishers, p. 42.

6. Amara Charles, 2011, *The Sexual Practices of Quodoushka*, Destiny Books.

7. Laddas, Whipple and Perry, op, cit, p.42.

8. Gary Schubach, 2001, "Urethral Expulsions During Sensual Arousal and Bladder Catheterization in Seven Human Females", *Electronic Journal of Human Sexuality*, 4.

9. S. Salama, F. Boitrelle, A. Gauquelin, L. Malagrida, N. Thiounn and P. Descaux, 2015, "Nature and origin of "squirting" in female sexuality." *Journal of Sexual Medicine*, 12.

10. Sheri Winston, op. cit.

11. Sharon Moalem and J. Reidenberg, 2009, "Does female ejaculation serve an antimicrobial purpose?" *Medical Hypotheses*. 73 (6):1069–71.

12. Sheila Kitzinger, op. cit, p. 218

13. Arthur Waley, (Translator), 1934, *The Way and Its Power: A Study of the Tao Te Ching and its Place in Chinese Thought*, Martino Fine Books, Chapter Six.

14. Philip Toshio Sudo, 2000, *Zen Sex*, San Francisco: Harper, p.79.

15. Catherine Blackledge, 2003, *The Story of V*, London: Phoenix.

Chapter Eight

1. Emily Nagoski, op. cit.

2. Sheri Winston, op. cit.

3. Nicole Daedone, 2011, *Slow Sex*, N.Y: Grand Central Publishing.

4. Mircea Eliade,1969, *Images and Symbols*, N.Y: Sheed and Ward, p.128.

5. Ibid.

6. Sylvia Brinton-Perera, op. cit, p.17–18.

Chapter Nine

1. Margaret Sheffield, 1989, *Life Blood: A New Image for Menstruation*. N.Y.: Alfred A. Knopf.

2. Penelope Shuttle and Peter Redgrove, 1978, *The Wise Wound*. London: Harper Collins, p. 29.

3. Lara Owen, 2008, *Her Blood is Gold*, U.K: Archive Publishing.

4. Virginia Beane Rutter, 1993, *Woman, Changing Woman*. New York: Harper Collins.

5. Ginger Collins Martire, 2006, *Menstrual Consciousness Development: An organic inquiry into the development of a psycho-spiritually rewarding menstrual relationship*. Doctoral dissertation, Institute of Transpersonal Psychology, Palo Alto, California. Unpublished manuscript.

6. Elizabeth Chubb, M.D. and Jane Knight, 1987, *Fertility*, David and Charles Publishers, p. 25.

7. Nelson Soucasaux, (date unknown), *How Menstruation Actually Occurs (at the Microscopic Level)*. Retrieved October 2017 from http://www.nelsonginecologia.med.br/localmechmenstre_engl.htm

8. Ina May Gaskin, 2003, *Ina May's Guide to Childbirth*. New York: Bantam Books.

9. Bruce Lipton, 2005, *The Biology of Belief: Unleashing the power of consciousness, matter and miracles*. Santa Rosa, California: Mountain of Love/Elite Books.

10. Martire, op. cit.

11. American Psychiatric Association, 2013, *Diagnostic and statistical manual of mental disorders (5th Ed.)*, Washington, DC: Author.

12. Progesterone also has anticonvulsant properties and has been used to chemically castrate perpetrators of violent sexual crimes.

13. Bonnie Horrigan, 1996, *Red Moon Passage: The power and wisdom of menopause*. London: Thorsons, p.114.

14. Lynne George, 1994, *A Female Cure for PMT*, Wellbeing Magazine No 67.

15. Owen, op. cit.

16. Judy Grahn, 1993, *Blood, Bread and Roses: How menstruation created the world*. Boston: Beacon Press.

17. Marija Gimbutas, 1989, *The Language of the Goddess*. New York: Thames and Hudson.

18. Elinor Gadon, 1989, *The Once and Future Goddess: A symbol for our time*. New York: Harper and Row.

19. Thomas Buckley and Alma Gottlieb (Eds.), 1988, *Blood Magic: The Anthropology of Menstruation*, Los Angeles: University of California Press, p. 7.

20. Jason Elias and Katherine Ketcham, 1995, *In The House of the Moon: Reclaiming the Feminine Spirit of Healing*, N. Y: Warner Books.

21. Brooke Medicine Eagle, 1991, *Buffalo Woman Comes Singing*. New York: Ballantine Books.

22. Shuttle and Redgrove, op. cit., p. 21.

Conclusion

1. Alexander Tsiaras and Barry Werth, 2002, *From Conception to Birth: A life unfolds*. London: Vermilion.

2. Philip Clayton, 2005, Theology and the physical sciences. In David Ford and Rachel Muers (Eds.), *The Modern Theologians: An introduction to Christian theology since 1918*, 3rd Edition, Oxford: Blackwell Publishing, p. 349.

3. Bill Plotkin, 2008, *Nature And The Human Soul: A roadmap to discovering our place in the world*. Sydney: Finch Publishing, p. 14.

Photo References

1. Egg cell – credit: Thierry Berrod, Mona Lisa Production/Science Photo Library. http://www.sciencephoto.com/

2. Earth – credit: Ryoota. https://www.istockphoto.com/au/stock-photos

3. Blastocyst with zona – credit: Jenny Nichols. https://wellcomecollection.org/works/rsmh4r6g?query=blastocyst+with+zona%3A+Jenny+Nichols

4. Hatching blastocyst – credit: K. Hardy. https://wellcomecollection.org/works/scfp2gf2?query=Hatching+blastocyst%3A+K.+Hardy

5. Cross-section through seminiferous tubule – credit: NIMR, Francis Crick Institute. https://wellcomecollection.org/works/fgaygsm9?query=sperm+in+seminiferous+tubule

6. Single sperm cell - credit: Steve Gschmeissner, Science Photo Library/Alamy Stock Photo. http://www.alamy.com/

7. Newly fertilised human egg - credit: Alan Handyside. https://wellcomecollection.org/works/bfsnpdbb?query=newly+fertilised+human+egg

8. Egg being fertilised by sperm - credit: Deco Images ll/Alamy Stock Photo. http://www.alamy.com/

9. Human embryo from IVF - credit: K. Hardy. https://wellcomecollection.org/works/ergc92jn?query=Human+embryo+from+IVF%3A+K.+Hardy

10. Internal view of a human embryo approx. 10 weeks - credit: Steve Allen Travel Photography/Alamy Stock Photo. http://www.alamy.com/

11. Cross section of Uterine Tube - credit: Steve Gschmeissner, Science Photo Library/Alamy Stock Photo, http://www.alamy.com/

12. Internal ecosystem of Uterine Tube - credit: Steve Gschmeissner, Science Photo Library/Alamy Stock Photo. http://www.alamy.com/

13. Inside the Uterine Tube - credit: Steve Gschmeissner, Science Photo Library. http://www.sciencephoto.com/

14. Coral reef – credit: mtec2. https://www.istockphoto.com/au/stock-photos

15. Endometrium – credit: Steve Gschmeissner - Science Photo Library. http://www.sciencephoto.com/

16. Woman with red paint on face – Le Pictorium/Alamy Stock Photo. http://www.alamy.com/

17. Carved Aboriginal cave art of female genitalia at Carnarvon Gorge, Australia – credit: Ray Wilson/Alamy Stock Photo. http://www.alamy.com/

18. Cave art limestone block with engraved vulva figures, La Ferrassie cave, Dordogne, France, c30,000 B.C. – credit: Granger Historical Picture Archive/Alamy Stock Photo. http://www.alamy.com/